4/6/79

To [illegible]

[illegible]

CRIME DOCTOR

DR. CHARLES P. LARSON, WORLD'S FOREMOST MEDICAL-DETECTIVE, REPORTS FROM HIS CRIME FILE

JOHN D. McCALLUM

The Writing Works, Inc.
Mercer Island, Washington

Gordon Soules Book Publishers
Vancouver, B.C., Canada

Library of Congress Cataloging in Publication Data

McCallum, John Dennis, 1924-
Crime Doctor.

1. Larson, Charles P., 1910- 2. Forensic pathologists—Washington (State)—Biography. 3. Forensic pathology—Cases, clinical reports, statistics. I. Title.
RA1025.L37M' 614'.19 78-16403
ISBN 0-916076-20-2

Published by The Writing Works, Inc.
7438 S.E. 40th Street
Mercer Island, WA 98040

ISBN: 0-916076-20-2 (Writing Works)
Library of Congress Catalog Card Number: 78-16403
Manufactured in the United States
Published in Canada by Gordon Soules Book Publishers
1118-355 Burrard Street
Vancouver, B.C., Canada V6C 2G8
ISBN: 0-919574-28-9 (Soules)

Foreword

By Frank P. Cleveland, M.D.
President, National Association of Medical Examiners, 1976-77

INFREQUENTLY, arising from the multitudes, there is a person, a leader, an innovator and dedicated worker who serves as a model and example to others in his field.

Such a man is Dr. Charles P. Larson, of Tacoma, Washington.

The scientific adventures and the investigative triumphs of Dr. Larson have been excellently captured in this book by author John D. McCallum for the edification of his countless friends, colleagues and the general public.

For the past 40 years, Dr. Larson has spent his life as a Forensic Pathologist. He has performed this public service as a private practitioner and has never held public office or a formal appointment in a law enforcement agency charged in the scientific investigation of death. His personal success in the scientific investigation of death is demonstrated through the media of case presentation.

Dr. Larson foresaw the need for education and development of scientific aids in the investigation of violent death and has spent much of his professional career in this endeavor. In 1937, Forensic Pathology was in its infancy in the United States. Dr. Larson, known far and wide as an expert in this field, carried the doctrine of scientific investigation of death to his community. Recognition of his capability in Forensic Pathology came from the College of American Pathologists where he served as president and also was chairman of the Forensic Pathology Committee. Similarly, he served as chairman of the Council of Forensic Pathology for the American Society of Clinical Pathologists and was one of the founders of the certification program in Forensic Pathology for the American Board of Pathology.

Forensic Pathology may be defined as that unique application of medical knowledge to the investigation of deaths to ascertain whether the death is natural, accidental, homicidal or suicidal. The medicolegal investigation of death encompasses a broad spectrum of activities. Dr. Larson—so-named the "Crime Doctor" years ago by former Tacoma prosecuting attorney Pat Steele—participates in the investigation of the scene where death occurs. From the examination of the death scene there will be derived evidence that will link the victim to a suspect. The evidence must first be recognized, secondly collected, identified and preserved, and then analyzed. The clothing of the victim is equally as important as the body of the victim, for from the clothing there will be derived proof of violence and recovery of trace evidence. Alterations of the clothing must be correlated with injuries upon the body of the victim. Thereafter, follows the examination of the body of the deceased person and from the post mortem examination of the body there is obtained a story of the victim's life and death, his health, disease and injury, and the cause of death. The data obtained by the Forensic Pathologist are factual, objective, unprejudiced and unbiased.

The factual information derived from the scene, the

clothing and the body allows the "Crime Doctor" to reach a valid medical conclusion as to the cause and manner of death. The same facts presented to a judge and jury permit the irrefutable identification, trial and conviction of the criminal who has perpetrated the crime. The Forensic Pathologist, Charles P. Larson, as an objective finder of fact, has applied his skills, knowledge, experience and intelligence to the discovery of deaths from violence and has assisted in the successful removal of the criminal from society.

A cosmopolitan, Dr. Larson was born in Eleva, Wisconsin, had his early education at Gonzaga University in Washington, obtained his medical degree from McGill University in Montreal, Quebec, and pursued specialty training in pathology at the University of Michigan and University of Oregon Medical Schools. His professional affiliations with Pathology Societies throughout the continental United States and international medical associations continue today.

Recognition of the qualities of leadership and of his dedication to this practice of pathology by his colleagues, eminate from his curriculum vitae. He has served as president of the major professional organizations in pathology. Service to his country as a colonel in the United States Army culminated in his being appointed pathologist for the War Crimes Investigating Team in the European Theater of Operation in 1945.

Dr. Larson was a founding member of the American Academy of Forensic Sciences in Chicago in 1948 and in 1966 was a founding member of the National Association of Medical Examiners. These two active national organizations provide assistance, guidance and leadership for those engaged in Forensic Pathology. The American Acedemy of Forensic Sciences has grown from a handful of founders to the present internationally active organization encompassing every discipline involved in the Criminal Justice System.

Scientific papers published in the Journal of Forensic

Sciences, founded by the American Academy of Forensic Sciences, are disseminated throughout the country to those practitioners in legal medicine and the related sciences. The Academy initiated the Forensic Science Foundation to develop new tools and investigate techniques for the medicolegal investigation of death.

The National Association of Medical Examiners has grown to an organization of approximately 400 physicians engaged in the investigation of death. With Dr. Larson's advice and support, this group has initiated a program for the improvement of medical examiners' and coroners' offices throughout the country by the development of standards for the medicolegal investigation of death. The scientific meetings of the National Association of Medical Examiners are dedicated to the improvement of our system of investigating deaths and provide assistance to those charged with the development of local and statewide systems. NAME has assisted in developing training programs for young physicians wishing to enter the field of Forensic Pathology.

Under Dr. Larson's leadership and stimulation, great strides have been made in providing qualified Forensic Pathologists to serve many communities in the United States. In the major metropolitan cities there is still a shortage of qualified persons in Forensic Pathology.

Dr. Larson's career as a father is, from a philosophical viewpoint, far more spectacular than that of the "Crime Doctor." His wife Margaret has directed the growth of seven children, four boys and three girls. Three of the boys are following medical careers in anesthesiology, pediatrics and rehabilitation medicine. The fourth son provides legal advice to his family. The girls have followed careers in education, social science and the arts.

As variety is essential to a full life, Dr. Larson has pursued an active interest in deep sea fishing and especially sought that salt-water delicacy, salmon. Physical condition, being an important element of an active medical practice, was maintained by early experience as an amateur boxer and later followed by a few professional bouts. Dr. Larson's interest and participation in sports are exemplified by his articles on deep sea fishing for the "Encyclopedia of Sports Medicine" and his performance as a referee in a world championship boxing match.

In addition to his professional activities, Dr. Larson has been active in his community. He has served as a member of the Washington State Athletic commission and was its chairman in 1958. He has been a member of Rotary International since 1940 and served as president of the Tacoma Athletic Commission in 1955. Being an avid sports fan, Dr. Larson was vice president of the National Boxing Association in 1960 and medical advisor to the National Wrestling Association. He was president of the National Boxing Association in 1961 and became the first president of the World Boxing Association in 1962.

Dr. Larson's career as a teacher began in 1939 as Professor of Anatomy and Histology at St. Martin's College in Lacey, Washington and continues today through his presentation of lectures and papers at professional society meetings and through his consultative services to various local and national institutions.

Dr. Charles P. Larson, student, father, scientist, physician, investigator, boxer and fisherman, has led an active life dedicated to a higher quality of medical practice in a highly specialized area, Forensic Pathology, and today stands forth as a symbol of excellence in medical practice and community involvement.

Dr. Larson having served his community well in many avenues of activity is now being honored and recognized through the biographical technique of displaying his professional prowess to the public.

January 12, 1978

To
Dr. Larson's
Wife, Margaret,
and
children

Contents

"Forensic pathologist. Primarily, pathology is the science of the origin, nature and the causes of diseases. But when you put the word forensic before it, you define the science as pertaining to, connected with, or used in courts of law, and you automatically include with the word diseases: poisoning, injuries and the destruction of parts of the human body incident to the crimes of assault, mayhem or homicide. A forensic pathologist is in effect a surgical detective—a crime doctor."

Dr. Charles P. Larson
1978

Crime Doctor

A 40-watt bulb overhead threw a pale light on the small doorway. The Merkle Hotel seemed to blend in with all the other dingy buildings on the block at 26th and Pacific; a shabby, run-down old structure of two stories, a miserable-looking place.

Dr. Charles P. Larson and Tacoma Police Chief Charles Zittle sat in the doctor's car a short distance away, their eyes glued on the hotel. Two squad cars were parked strategically behind them, waiting for a signal. Dr. Larson looked at his wristwatch. "Five more minutes and we're going in," he told Zittle. He slumped down in his seat and waited.

Dr. Larson was 46 at the time, broad of shoulder, flat-gutted, with a fine, steady cock to his chin. He was part forensic pathologist, part detective, with ice for nerves. Pat Steele, the county prosecutor, had dubbed him the "Crime Doctor" in 1947—and the nickname stuck.

The street was quite dark. It was one of those nights that late spring is supposed to be for, but Dr. Larson did not like it at all. He shifted in his seat, sucked at a cigarette.

"We've got plenty of security," Chief Zittle reminded him. "Don't worry, Charley, everything will be fine."

"We cannot afford to guess wrong," Dr. Larson said. "We told her we'd give her 10 minutes, and then we're going in." He checked his watch again. Three more minutes.

The object of his concern was Patty Marshall (not her real name), a recent graduate of the University of Puget Sound and the first female police officer in Tacoma to cover a regular beat. She had volunteered to work undercover, posing as a pregnant woman seeking an abortion. Marjorie Smith, operating out of the Merkle, ran the busiest abortion mill in the county.

Marjorie Smith. There was the smell of sin about her. Her annual gross income was up around $500,000, easy. She was a tough old dame—big, foul-mouthed, with the disposition of a fighting cock. Her illegal profession rankled Dr. Larson and he, as well as Chief Zittle, wanted her busted and out of circulation. They had devised a flawless plan, or so they hoped. It went like this:

The day before the raid, Patty went to the Merkle and made a $100 deposit with Ms. Smith. The going rate was $200. Patty promised to pay the balance the next night when she came in for the operation. It was urgent, she told Smith, that she have the abortion as soon as possible, because she was already six weeks along. (Actually, she wasn't pregnant at all.)

On the night of her appointment, Patty sat in the car with Dr. Larson and Chief Zittle, listening to final instructions. She was a good-looking woman, youngish, well-groomed and attractively dressed. There was nothing to indicate that she was a cop.

"We'll be timing it right on the nose," Chief Zittle told her. "We're coming in *exactly* 10 minutes after you step through the front door."

Dr. Larson nodded. "That's just enough time for you to pay her, get up on the table and have your legs ready—and for the abortion to begin," Dr. Larson said.

Patty smiled. She was a gutsy gal.

"Don't be late," she said.

Chief Zittle then gave her $100 in small bills. The money was marked with a fluorescent material for identification purposes.

Dr. Larson looked at his watch again. One more minute. It was tough, he thought, to be waiting and wondering about Patrolwoman Marshall and trying to read her mind from a distance. And if she got hurt, he would never forgive himself for not having been at the scene in time.

Finally, he said to the Chief, "All right, Chuck, that's it. The 10 minutes are up. Let's go."

Then there was a flurry of movement; the front door caving in from brute force, and yelling and obscenities (by Ms. Smith) and Patty asking Dr. Larson, "What kept you?" That had been cutting it pretty close, at that. Two more minutes and Ms. Smith would have started giving an unpregnant woman an abortion!

Today, Dr. Larson can still recall the details: "We timed our arrival right on the button," he says. "We smashed through the door just as Smith was ready to start. That was critical. Patty had lots of nerve to go in there and submit to an abortion—when she wasn't even pregnant. The minute we came in, Smith knew what we were there for. I never heard such vile language in all my life. She could cuss worse than a Missouri muleskinner. She was especially mad at Patty. We took the marked money from her, and, of course, we had her stone cold.

"Marjorie Smith's abortion clinic was very unsanitary. The floors were dirty—no wonder there was so much infection among her clients—and she had no means of properly sterilizing her equipment. She had no medical training whatsoever. This had led to several deaths. The way she worked was to put her patients to bed after spreading newspapers on it. There was a ward with four beds in it. She had an old gynecological table that must have been about 1910 vintage. She had rubber drainage pads that the patient placed her butt on, and when the blood started squirting, everything ran down on the floor. I proved she'd been doing abortions by simply going around the edges of the baseboard with a pen knife and scraping material off it. Later, in my lab, I made sections of those scrapings and found pieces of placental and decidual tissues from many different women who'd been aborted there. The place never had been decently cleaned, one reason for all those infections. The only sterilizing equipment Smith had was an old hotwater sterilizer, which, of course, was totally inadequate because it didn't kill any of the real virulent organisms which can cause infectious hepatitis and all sorts of diseases.

"The only lamp she had was a goose-neck office lamp. There were no operating lights. Anybody can buy this old secondhand equipment from a medical supply house; credentials are not necessary. There's a hell of a profit in surgical equipment. All told, Marjorie Smith's investment wasn't worth more than $500—yet she was netting thousands of dollars a month. At $200 per patient, she had eight beds, and, doubling production, I figured she was performing up to 16 abortions a day. She didn't keep anybody overnight. That would have been bad for business. She kept no records, because she would have had to pay taxes on a whopping income, if the IRS had nailed her. In those days, abortions were a hush-hush business. They were carried on in secret. If a woman had an abortion, she didn't go around telling the world about it. She simply paid the fee and said nothing. And so people like Marjorie Smith got rich.

"What did the courts do to her? She was tried and convicted on two counts: (1) for performing an illegal abortion, and (2) manslaughter. She was sent to prison—but it was a relatively *light* sentence. They should have thrown the key away."

It is a fact of modern society that before you die, you *may* commit murder, you stand a chance of being accused of committing murder, and a very good chance, in the world's present jungle culture, of *being* murdered.

In any of these events, a good man to have on your side would be Dr. Larson; a good man because, as a forensic pathologist (an M.D. who specializes in crime-oriented autopsies), he usually helps law enforcement authorities get their man. Once, a year-long survey of his triumphs vs. his failures was conducted, and it revealed that of the more than 30 homicides brought to him during those 12 months, 87 percent of them were solved. This, as opposed to the less than 35 percent for all of the police forces the world around.

If you opt for committing murder and want to get away with it, advises Dr. Larson, do it in hot blood on the spur of the moment, because unless you kill an old friend, murders done in quick flares of passion are harder to solve than carefully planned murders. Intricately planned homicides are the products of abnormal minds that are prone to make mistakes—that have blind spots—that overplay the action. But, then, if they were normal, they would not at the last moment go through with it.

A slight mistake is all that Dr. Larson ever needs; blonde hair on the jacket sleeve of a black-haired man and gray stains on his trousers that in the crime lab turn out to be smears of human brain tissue, for example.

To be wrongfully accused of murder is not so hard to come by as you might think. In fact, a great many people have walked right into it, as casually as you please—or as stupidly. Some of those people are undoubtedly still doing time. One, of record, isn't. What he did was to leave his bloody footprints all around a body that had ceased violently to be active, and all around the adjacent area as well.

The local police didn't have to look twice. As soon as they looked once, they had their "killer." The Washington state patrolman happened on the scene first. When Dr. Larson straightened that one out, he strongly suggested that the patrolman take a course in Homicide Investigative Procedure.

"When they call me," Dr. Larson says, "the first thing I insist on, before I move in, is that they seal the whole area off and put tight security on it. I can't work if somebody has messed up the evidence before I get there."

In the matter of having your own life brought to its end by a murderer, "the chances are extremely good," according to Dr. Larson, "because we have only 200,000 trained policemen in a country of 217,000,000 people whose mixed cultures and minority belligerence have made a hobby of homicide in certain sections and big business of it in others."

In Las Vegas, the last checkout found the price of a killing to be holding steady at about $50, because there is the whole desert around to lay bodies out on and they are rarely found.

"If you are going to be killed, and you want your killer caught, have a close friend knock you off," Dr. Larson points out. "Because an impersonal, out-of-town paid gun leaves damned little spoor. The hit man flies in, has somebody finger you, pockets the price, squeezes off and flies out again. No other connection with you at all except the money. No motive whatever—beyond the money. Two total strangers—you and your killer. No intertwining of lives to be carefully unwoven until the motive and the murderer stand sharply outlined against the white light of justice. That is the one killer the police fear—the paid gun—because he usually gets away with murder."

Here is a very easy way to get yourself accused of murder. Your wife's out of town and you don't care too much about her even when she's in town. So you go to a tavern for a few beers and you pick up a girl with yes eyes. You take her home and have a few more drinks with her until she begins to look like one of those centerspread girls. The next morning you reach out for her with a matinee in mind and find her body as cold and clammy as a haunch of veal. Her eyes are open, but they don't see you. Nor are they ever going to see anyone or anything ever again.

Now, a No. 9 hangover is not the best equipment to face a situation of this kind with, but after a fashion you do face it (as did the Taxpayer to whom this actually happened). For openers, you reluctantly call the police.

While awaiting their arrival, bits and pieces of the lost weekend begin to filter back through the alcoholic fog, but for the life of you (and your life may well be the price) you cannot remember how the woman ceased to be alive.

But the police start right in probing for reasons. "How did the body come by so many bruises? She looks as if she played four quarters against the Green Bay Packers—both ways!"

A vignette flashes back of the dead woman's deciding that she was the Statue of Liberty, and of her going up the stairs, wrapped in a sheet, to hold a lighted candle above her head at the top.

"She fell down stairs a lot."

"What do you mean a lot?"

"Everytime she went upstairs, she fell down."

"You better get a lawyer, fellow."

They took the body down for a routine autopsy, and a part of the report was that one blow it had sustained was massive enough to separate the brain from the spinal cord. They booked the Taxpayer on suspicion of murder. *Strong* suspicion.

The defense attorney retained by the suspect to fight for his life called in Dr. Larson. As he absolutely *loathes* doing, Dr. Larson came in late on the case, after everybody else had been wading through the evidence up to their knees.

Dr. Larson is a six-foot tall, quiet man with twinkling eyes, a warm sense of humor, who is alive to living—probably because his profession is making dead people *talk*—and he has never been known to raise his voice in the process.

On the body of this dead woman, Dr. Larson asked authority to perform another autopsy *himself*, a postmortem if you will. He found in the process that the bruises she had sustained were not all inflicted at the same time; that if they were a result of falling down stairs, which they well could have been, she had possibly played Statue of Liberty quite a few times on different days during the last week she and the suspect had been sleeping together.

Dr. Larson found that the woman's brain had *not* been severed from the spinal cord by a blow but by inept surgery on the part of the general practitioner who had been called in by the coroner to perform the original autopsy.

"This is one of the reasons that people can get away with murder in the United States," Dr. Larson said. "A coroner generally is an elected or appointed politician who in most communities does not have to have any specialized training of any kind. He has an office and the title and the authority to play around at cops and robbers when someone buys the farm but very little else. If he wants an autopsy performed, he throws the fee to a friend who is an M.D., who by the very fact that he picks up work of that kind is not necessarily too well qualified or experienced professionally."

For years Dr. Larson has continually pointed out that a corps of about 1,500 highly specialized autopsy surgeons—trained for postmortem surgery as carefully as physicians train for any other specialty—would cut the number of people who "get away with murder" today to practically zero tomorrow; for there are very few dead bodies that, under competent investigative procedures, will fail to "tell" how they came to die. As it is, there are probably less than 200 full time forensic pathologists in the whole country.

"It is most difficult to get recruits," Dr. Larson says. "By the very nature of the medical profession, doctors are trained to *save* lives—not to work with dead ones."

With the Statue-of-Liberty woman, as soon as Dr. Larson had found out what it was that she had *not* died of, he went after the cause of her death through all of the bungled work of the first autopsy. It was still there, the cause of her death, and Dr. Larson found it—a very common cause of the deaths of drunks—food in her throat that she had choked upon. She had, drunk, gotten up to eat and, still chewing, laid down again beside her snoring companion and, in the prone position, being unable to swallow freely, she choked to death.

By such simple misadventures, we sometimes die. And by such matter-of-fact discovery of the real cause of death, those people who have been picked up on suspicion of murder are exonerated. To face an irate wife?

Not in this case, for the police, having made a mistake, agreed to keep Mr. Taxpayer's wife out of it when she came back to town. So possibly he *did* get away with murder.

When the police of any city are successful in running down a criminal, the public seems to take it very much for granted. The reason being, I suppose, that in whodunits, on television and in the movies, the detective always solves the mystery.

In real life he doesn't. He fails about as often as he succeeds. Perhaps oftener. When he fails, the citizenry screams at him, reviles him, makes fun of him.

How dare he fail! He's got 200 men to run down a laundry mark for him; 150 more to comb a suberb for a green paint nerf on the fence post into a driveway. But still he can fail, and does.

With homicide there is a cut-and-dried formula. The procedure, theoretically, is so very simple. Examine, photograph, diagram the scene of the crime without disturbing it. Study the autopsy surgeon's report. This produces *when, where* and *how.* All that is needed now is the motive—*why.* Determine that and it *should* lead to *who.*

But it doesn't always lead to anything.

Law enforcement is an eternal defensive war. The attacking force consists of those men and women and sometimes children who congenitally are unable to live within the law; or who, balancing the penalty against their personal wants, decide to break the law; or who, in crisis, are unable to control themselves *within* the law.

In a defensive posture against such people stand the police forces of the world—the constant firing line ever since the Code of Hammurabi was established at the beginning of written history with Babylonian soldiers to enforce it. Constant warriors, the police, who alone make it possible for man to live in a continuing pattern of comparative safety. Hate the cop or respect the cop, but you cannot live without him, for when you try, the criminal at once takes over, because that is the nature of man. He will not live at peace with himself. He has to hire a policeman to make him. The police win and the police lose in individual cases, but the overall result is still victory. If it were not so, the world by now would be nothing but an anarchic free-for-all.

"If psychiatrists dug into the high emotional level that police work calls for at times, it would drive them up the wall," Dr. Larson was saying. "And if a man tried to be an expert in all the things that a policeman has to do in a normal day's work, it would take him 50 years of schooling."

I once spent a day riding with two police squadcar men in Manhattan. They had invited me along for a firsthand glimpse of what their professional lives were all about. "One shift with us and you'll have enough material for six stories," they said.

Rocco and Webster, I will call them. We sat in their police car on lower Broadway listening to the dispatcher's staccato. The radio never let up. With one ear they listened. New York City's troubles.

"Two women fighting over a lost garbage can..."

"That's us," and Rocco rolled the car. Webster located the garbage can and they left the women laughing.

"Baby dying," and the squadcar rolled. They alerted Community Hospital, and when they saw the mother at the curb, Rocco slowed while Webster took the baby on the fly. They floor-boarded to the hospital, Code Three. A doctor stood in Emergency. He ran with the baby. Two years old with a jagged splinter of glass in her neck—but they saved her. *They saved that baby.*

The car radio crackled on. "Suspected burglary," and the squadcar rolled. A woman stuttering with fear. She showed Webster the forced window. They went into the house, guns drawn, and found the burglar—the woman's teenage son, asleep in bed. He had forgotten his key.

The radio again—"Bank robbery in progress," and the car rolled again—three minutes away from the sharpest gunfight of the year. At 4 o'clock, Rocco died in surgery.

Later that night at dinner, Webster's wife said, "Did you have a good day, Honey?" And Webster said, "I guess so—what's for dinner?" He did not want to ruin her meal. Later, he would tell her about Rocco. And still later, in bed, he would stare at the ceiling, sleepless, facing it—that his partner was dead—that his laughter was forever gone into silence.

Dr. Larson:

"The first time I realized the kind of life I had *really* committed myself to was when I got a letter from an inmate at the state pen vowing he was going to kill me when he got out. I had helped to convict him. I guess I have had at least a dozen threats on my life. But in spite of some hairy moments, I can truthfully say that nothing that ever happened to me in my whole career has ever made me wish that I had chosen any other way of life. The going never gets so tough, investigation work never gets so baffling or the conditions of the eternal chase so frustrating that I have ever wanted to turn back. In a lot of ways I'm probably like that happy policeman who is 80 percent of any force. Without that 80 percent you couldn't have a police force. He likes his job. He is dedicated to his job. He is satisfied with the conditions of his job. In many, many cases he doesn't particularly scrabble full-out for promotion. He has a wife and kids usually, and with today's pay scales he can have a good way of life.

"I would say that the best policeman is the same kind of a man as a good truck driver. The good truck driver is a sober man, a trustworthy man, well-grounded in the operation and routine maintenance of the vehicle he drives. He is a man experienced and self-schooled in keeping schedules and in carrying out commitments. On the highways he sets the example of the finest type of driving. He keeps himself fit for back-breaking schedules, which are routine with him, and for the crises he must meet eternally without any warning. He is a truck driver because he *wants* to be a truck driver, because he takes pride in driving his truck, because *he likes driving a truck.*

"This is not to say that policemen lack ambition, because there is a challenge to police work that *inspires* ambition. Without those policemen who meet this challenge by acquiring special skills, experience and knowledge beyond the routine of the patrol car, there could be no organized police forces and no continuing effort toward crime suppression. Because there are these challenges, the same challenges that make top-flight diagnosticians out of some doctors, internationally-respected jurists out of some lawyers, consultants in far countries out of some engineers, there are no limits in the police profession to which a man can aspire."

The Crime Doctor

A deliberate selling title, if you will—but that is what his colleagues in the crime-bustin' world call him. The telephone will ring at Tacoma General Hospital, and someone in London or Atlanta or New South Wales or Alaska will ask to speak to the "Crime Doctor"—and the call is put through to the Pathology Lab, on the street floor next to Emergency, to Dr. Charles P. Larson. For 40 years his services have been in demand by police authorities all over the world. There is no obscure secret involved. No man can build a stronghold that another man cannot capture. No man can commit murder without leaving spoor that a properly trained investigator cannot follow, until it leads to the killer.

I have known Dr. Larson for about 20 years. He has it—the tools of his trade—an infallible memory, a sleepless curiosity, bulldog tenacity.

One of the most infamous criminal cases of the 1950s involved Dr. Sam Sheppard, who was accused of bludgeoning his wife to death in Cleveland. Dr. Larson entered the investigation about a year after the homicide and prior to the final conviction.

"This was through a phone call I received from one of Dr. Sam's defense attorneys," Dr. Larson said. "He wanted to know if I'd be willing to reinvestigate some of the scientific facts that he knew were going to come up in court during the trial. I told him I'd do it if he'd pay my expenses, which he did. So I made a brief investigation of the incidents and scientific data gathered by the prosecution. I knew the coroner assigned to the case—Dr. Samuel Gerber, a very well-known medical legal expert—and I felt that the work which had been done in the original investigation of the case on the scene and in the crime lab was adequate, excellent and impeccable. In my own search I did not find anything which I could use to aid the defense of Dr. Sheppard—and so advised his defense attorney. On the basis of that, I was never called to testify.

"It wasn't my place to decide whether or not Dr. Sam was guilty, but I had learned enough during my brief investigation of the facts that I most certainly couldn't help him. I found nothing to *prove* his innocence. The jury decided he was guilty, and that was good enough for me."

At the Sheppard retrial a Dr. Kirk was called in to testify. He was a prominent criminologist from the University of California and author of a book dealing with investigation of physical evidence. He testified that there had been, actually, *two* different types of "O" blood at the murder scene.

"As far as I am concerned, that's an *impossibility,"* Dr. Larson said, in reviewing the case for me. "There are not two types of 'O' blood. There is only one type of 'O' blood—and that's 'O' blood. But Dr. Kirk testified there were two different people involved who had 'O' blood, on a basis of the different titres of the agglutins in the dried blood spots. But it's a known fact, depending on what blood dries on—whether it's a firm, hard surface, wood, metal, cloth, cement, etc.—that the titre of known agglutins and agglutinogens can vary tremendously, even though the blood is all from the same person. Therefore, I was convinced that Dr. Kirk's testimony was totally unethical and even untrue. However, on the basis of his testimony, Dr. Sheppard got a new trial and was eventually released from prison—to take up a new career as a professional wrestler, of all things.

"Dr. Kirk was knowledgeable enough to realize he didn't tell the whole truth under oath; he *knew* he was treading on a very thin line between what was possible and what was impossible. I was so upset by him that I and several other experts in the field of forensic pathology testified against him at an ethics meeting of the American Academy of Forensic Pathologists—and his membership was suspended on the basis of our testimony."

There was one case Dr. Larson got involved in quite by accident. It came about by his guest appearance on Earl Stanley Gardner's old TV program, "The Court of Last Resort." Afterward, there was a flood of mail, appealing to Dr. Larson for help. A mother in San Francisco wrote that her son was serving life in San Quentin on a first-degree murder charge. He had already spent two years there, she wrote. "Deep in my heart," the letter read, "I know he didn't do it." She added that she was employed as a stenographer, that she did not have much money and would be able to afford only $15 a month if Dr. Larson would take the case. "But I will pay you for as long as I live," she stated.

The mother's letter piqued Dr. Larson's interest.

He phoned her and agreed to reinvestigate the facts. He told her it was vital that she send him a copy of a letter written by a well-known pathologist who had signed the autopsy report and had testified at the trial of her son—in spite of the fact that the actual autopsy had been performed by a resident of his and not by himself personally. Following Dr. Larson's instructions, the mother, at considerable cost to herself, secured a transcription of the medical testimony as it had been given in court. The transcription indicated to Dr. Larson that the conviction was based largely on scientific medical evidence and not on other facts of the case. In studying the transcript and weighing it against what the mother had told him, it seemed to Dr. Larson that there were possible errors in the medical testimony.

Dr. Larson:

"The key to the whole case in the medical testimony was the fact that the pathologist who testified in court stated that the deceased had been stabbed several times with a long butcher knife. All these stabs, he said, were through one wound in the chest, but that the knife was jerked partially out and moved in different directions, up and down and sideways, several times, producing several injuries in both the chest and abdomen. The entrance stab wound was in the fourth left intercostal space anteriorly.

"It occurred to me that I should look up in a cross-sectional anatomy book and see if I could determine whether all of these wounds of different organs as described in the autopsy protocol could have been produced by a single stab wound. The reason for this was that the son's testimony stated that he and his roommate (male) had gone out the night before the killing and gotten drunk. Both boys were the same age.

"Now, the roommate had been depressed. A month earlier he'd shot himself in the foot in an abortive attempt at suicide and was still wearing a cast. Both boys awoke the next morning with hangovers. The one boy, the accused, got up first to make breakfast. While he was in the kitchen, his roommate shouted from the bedroom suddenly, 'Gimme a butcher knife! I'm gonna kill myself!' Thinking it was only a gag, and going along with it, the accused tossed him a butcher knife. It landed at the foot of the bed. The roommate grabbed it and plunged the knife into his chest.

"In court, the doctor refuted that it happened that way. He claimed that the blade had been moved in an up-and-down-and-sideways direction several times, causing multiple wounds to various organs. The organs he described included the tip of the lower lobe of the right lung, a buttonhole through-and-through wound, a buttonhole through-and-through wound in the tip of the right ventricle of the heart, a through-and-through wound of the diaphragm, a penetrating wound to the liver, a penetrating wound to the stomach that went through and through, and a penetrating wound of the duodenum.

"On the basis of all these injuries, he postulated that the knife had been moved several times after it had been plunged into the body. At first, I didn't know how to solve this, even with cross-sectional anatomy, which indicated that possibly all those wounds to different organs had been inflicted by a single knife wound. I concluded there was no way to solve the mystery except to *stab human bodies!*

"To prove my theory, I stabbed the next 30 bodies which I autopsied. They were all dead individuals, of course; I was going to cut them open anyway. So the fact that I stabbed them made no difference. I stabbed them with a butcher knife which was identical with the one described in the case—the same length, the same blade width, the same sharpness. I found that in more than 50 percent of the cases in which I made a single through-and-through stab wound in the chest, every single injury described in court by the pathologist was produced."

That cinched it. Dr. Larson had broken the case wide open. He testified at a hearing by the California State Board of Parole, provided them and Governor Edmund Brown with written reports. Result: The boy won his freedom from San Quentin.

What sort of man is Dr. Larson?

He is this sort of man—he never sent the mother a bill. "Considering what she and her son had been through," he said, "and taking their financial situation into account, I preferred to charge that one up to experience."

His Chief in the Army said to him once: "Colonel, you think like a cop, you work like a cop and there are even times when you smell like a cop!"

Dr. Larson grinned.

"You run that down for a make, sir, and you'll probably find it's because I've worked with cops most of my life."

Dr. Larson is by no means the only white-coat who uses a test tube like a butterfly net to capture criminals. There are toxicologists who can sniff a poisoning halfway across town and anthropologists who read bones as handily as most people peruse the morning paper. Any pathologist worth his sodium chloride can reconstruct for you a fine murder scene by performing a postmortem. Dr. Larson, though, is a master at all these macabre chores, and more, mainly because, unlike most of his colleagues in the scientific-sleuthing arts, he thinks of himself as a detective as well as a scientist.

Frequently he has helped solve riddles in which his medical background has been of little or no use and, through a sort of on-the-job training, he has become wise enough to be accepted by courts as an expert on such diverse subjects as firearms identification and handwriting.

In a forgery case some years ago the Larson testimony was so skillful on behalf of the prosecutor that a handwriting expert hired by the defense clomped out of the courtroom without ever speaking up.

As a free-lancing crime doctor, he works the way any other physician or any lawyer would do, on a fee-for-service basis available either to the defense or to the police. Most often, quite naturally, it is the law side which summons him. One day, the police department of Olympia, Washington, called him. The caller said Dr. Larson should hurry on down there because he *thought* a woman was dead. This turned out to be a somewhat conservative summary of the situation. Alice Imlay was very much dead. Mrs. Imlay, 80, had been living in an orderly frame house on an Olympia street lined with great shade trees in a quiet, middle-class part of town.

When Dr. Larson arrived on the scene and first saw the victim, she reposed on the floor of her second-story bedroom. Besides being raped, she had been slugged, beaten and punctured numerous times with a knife. Apparently as an afterthought, or simply because times were tough, her killer also had attempted to take a big *bite* out of Grandmother Imlay. Imprinted in her left breast was a neat row of teeth marks near the nipple. The right nipple had been eaten off. The French call that *manger la nipple.* To Dr. Larson this was a gesture of cooperation on the murderer's part practically like leaving a signed note saying where he might be reached later.

Those teeth marks got his adrenalin flowing, like a prospector whose Geiger counter starts chattering. As he combed the room, he then found what he considered at the time a perfect signpost to at least the *kind* of person who might bite Mrs. Imlay. What he found on the floor was a bloody heel print, not just an ordinary print, but the outline of a small, narrow, Cuban-type heel. Considerable film was devoted to it by Ken Ollar, a photographer who frequently was at Dr. Larson's side to record for posterity and for juries the scenes of his friend's triumphs of mind over murder.

"I'm thinking of suspects in terms of that heel," Dr. Larson said, staring down at the print. "I'm thinking of cowboys, zoot suiters, motorcyclists. All of those people wear that kind of shoe or boot."

"The kid next door rides a motorcycle," one of the policemen helpfully put in.

"What kid?" snapped Dr. Larson.

"The Howdeshell boy. It was his mother who called us—though it was odd she hadn't seen the old lady around. Oh, but the boy's got an airtight alibi. We checked it out. Funny thing, though, he was outside when we got here and kept saying, 'You'll find lits of my fingerprints in there. I do her odd jobs.'"

"Yeah," said Dr. Larson. "Funny thing."

After he had carefully scrutinized every square inch of the Imlay house and every pore of the Imlay remains, Dr. Larson walked outside, lit a cigarette and stood on the sidewalk, chatting with the bluecoats. He kept staring wistfully at the house next door.

"Damn it, Doctor, we can't go back in there," pleaded one of the officers. "That's a respectable family. Never any trouble."

"I'd like to *see* him anyway," Dr. Larson replied. "I've got a hunch."

A couple of policemen followed him into the Howdeshell house. The boy's name was Roy. He was 18, clean-cut, calm and polite, even helpful.

"Roy's never owned any motorcycling boots," said his mother. A search of the house turned up none. But one of the officers picked a tiny object off the floor in Roy's bedroom. He handed it to Dr. Larson. "Probably nothing. Just a button," he said. He was right. It was only a plain gray button from a sports shirt. As Dr. Larson rolled the button over between his thumb and finger and peered at it, though, he noticed a pin-point-sized brown stain in one of the thread holes. "Bring Roy along," he told the officer. "I want to see what this is."

At the Olympia branch lab he maintained, Dr. Larson put the button through tests and found, just as he suspected, that the speck was a blood-stain. He couldn't prove it was Mrs. Imlay's blood. But it was her type and not Roy's.

Dr. Larson began to study scrapings from beneath Roy's fingernails, and Ken Ollar, the versatile photographer, was washing the boy's hair over a basin looking for more blood—which they found both in the head hair and under the foreskin of his penis. They were still at it when Roy suddenly blurted, "Okay—okay! I did it!" A short sentence that was to cost him a long one—life.

Dr. Larson didn't need the dental report which showed Roy's teeth matched the marks on widow Imlay. And it was days before they found out who wore those odd-shaped heels. (It was a state patrolman who'd reached the scene first.)

"That print was a red herring, all right," Dr. Larson told the press later. "But you'll have to admit it led us in the right direction. Prints usually do because even when a heel is new, it's unlike any other. No two human 'heels' are alike, either."

After typing up tapes of interviews I had with Dr. Larson for this book, my secretary, Audrey E. Neil, asked me, "My god—do people like Dr. Larson actually *live* outside of books?" They do—and around such men books such as this are written.

In This Corner: "Kid Philips"

THE Roaring Twenties suited young Charles Philip Larson perfectly. It was an age of superlatives. Everything that was done right was done more right and bigger than ever. The same applied to everything that was done wrong. Hoodlums no longer fought each other with stones and bats. Now they took each other for a one-way ride in an automobile.

It was an era of exaggeration, too. Men who had been casual drinkers now had to get drunk. Women were not satisfied with the role of attracting the male to marriage and making a home for him. They had to be his equal on the public forum, in politics and in bed. It was also a time of high finance. A smart man saved his money and acquired $25,000; a clever one played the market and made a million. In defiance of law, men made alcohol in cellar distilleries, bottled beer and sold it with an eye against a slot in the door. Young ladies cut their hair, shortened their dresses, drank gin, danced the Charleston and read Dr. Warner Fabian's *Flaming Youth.*

There were flagpole sitters, cross-country walkers, marathon dancers and the beginning of air-mail flights from New York to San Francisco. Everybody was trying to make Ripley's "Believe It Or Not." Young Larson, 17, did. He made a hole-in-one the first time he played golf. He quit the game after that, saying "I can't improve on that."

An insurance company booklet described Moses as "one of the greatest salesmen and real-estate promoters that ever lived," and Jesus Christ was called "the founder of modern business."

They called it the "era of wonderful nonsense," and nowhere was the hysteria more boisterous or the screaming louder than in sports. Throwing off its bush-league trappings, sports suddenly erupted in the 1920s as big business and lavish entertainment. The decade witnessed the first million-dollar prizefight and World Series, and produced more vital, vibrant performers than any other decade in the chronicles of athletics. Every sport had a dominant personality who attracted and held public attention, for this was the era of Ty Cobb, still slashing into third, his spikes aglimmer; Babe Ruth standing at the plate on his thin, matchstick ankles, slowly waving his bludgeon like a cobra poised to strike; Big Bill Tilden banging his unreturnable cannonball service across the net; Bobby Jones, waving to cheering thousands—after winning the golf championships of Great Britain—as he received a ticker-tape reception down Broadway, an event previously reserved only for visiting royalty and transatlantic aviators; the death wagons roaring around the Indianapolis speedway track at 125 miles per hour; Paavo Nurmi dog-trotting around the running track in a steady, devasting assault upon Time.

The Jazz Age.

The Golden Decade.

The Roaring Twenties.

Whatever you called it, it was the last big spree between World Wars, marking a national rite of passage, a maudlin farewell to the innocence and hope of a childhood now irrevocably gone. And it was more than just a coincidence that when this age found its poet, F. Scott Fitzgerald would write longingly of the pads worn for a day on the football fields of Princeton.

For young Charley Larson, who was born on August 15, 1910 in Eleva, Wisconsin—which took its name from the first five letters of the word elevator, at the fifth letter of which some long forgotten sign painter stopped painting a trackside grain elevator and walked off the job—the 1920s were largely gold and cheering crowds and gallant heroes of the prize ring. *Boxing*—that was his cup of tea.

After the Larsons moved to Spokane, where Charley's father was president of the Farmers and Mechanics Bank, the boy joined the YMCA and made the boxing team. At 13, he put on the gloves for the first time—and, at 16, he had his first professional fight. The way that came about was this:

"I fought numerous amateur bouts and won most of them," Dr. Larson recalls. "I was a good amateur welterweight, was never KO'd. I was big for my age, 6 feet tall and 147 pounds. Leo Lompski, the old heavyweight contender, used to visit the Y and gave us lessons. One of those who sparred with me was Albert Rosellini—later our governor. In 1926, when I was 16, this promoter saw me sparring in the gym at the Y. He said, 'How'd you like to make $100 fighting in one of the prelims?' The main event was Lompski vs. Fred Lenhart, a great matchup. I said, 'Who do I have to *kill*?' And the promoter said, 'Don't worry, Son. I'll talk to your opponent and he'll carry you.' So he nicknamed me 'Kid Philips'—after my middle name —and I agreed to the terms."

The opponent was a 32-year-old black, a veteran. But his experience did not dim Charley's self-confidence one bit. At the opening bell, he waded into the old pro with leather flying in all directions and tattooed him good. In the clinches his opponent advised him to slow down. "Take it easy, boy," the black said. "Pace yourself. You're going to punch yourself out. There's still five rounds to go."

They were in the fourth round, when the black fighter said, "Well, boy, this is where I'm going to have to put you to sleep. I hope I don't hurt you."

Then the lights went out. The next thing Charley remembered he was flat on his back in the dressing room, being revived.

"I'd opened and closed in one," Dr. Larson smiled, borrowing an old vaudeville expression. "That ended my professional boxing aspirations."

But it didn't end his connection with boxing. In 1961, he served as president of the National Boxing Association; in 1962, he was elected Founding President of the World Boxing Association.

"When I was a young man growing up in Spokane," Dr. Larson told me, "my heroes were Jack Dempsey and Gene Tunney. I was so crazy about the prize ring that I even hitchhiked to Shelby, Montana, to watch Dempsey and Tommy Gibbons go 15 rounds, the only one of Dempsey's championship fights to go the distance. I crawled under the fence to get in.

"I remember still the gloom hanging over Spokane like dense fog the morning after Tunney beat Dempsey in 1926. I was then in my first year of college at Gonzaga University—I was three classes behind Bing Crosby—and I had a part-time job in the insurance department of the *Spokesman-Review*, the morning paper. The only form of radio we had to follow the fight in those days was old-fashioned crystal sets with earphones. I didn't get to hear the fight. Newspapers were still the No. 1 way for Americans to get their news, and I arranged with the fellows down in the pressroom to give me the first bundles of the early edition, banner-lining the fight story on page one. Then I went out and hired 15 kids to sell papers for me. You should have been there. Hot off the press, we raced up and down the main streets of Spokane hawking those papers.

The customers gobbled them up like hot cakes, eager to read the round-by-round details of Tunney's stunning upset of the old champ. Some of the fans were in such a frenzy to 'read all about it,' they shelled out $1 for the paper. We sold more than 3,000 copies within the first hour after hitting the streets. I cleaned up. I'll always be grateful to Dempsey and Tunney for helping me earn money for my schooling. Now, do you understand why I've always had such a soft spot in my heart for prizefighting?"

Over the years, Dr. Larson has examined numerous autopsy reports relating to boxing fatalities. His exhaustive research has included a large number of reports from the New York Medical Examiner's Office, as well as many other state medical examiners' and coroners' offices in the United States; a similar number came from foreign countries, principally European. Analysis of these autopsy studies have indicated that the main cause of death in almost all cases was subarachnoid hemorrhage.

"This is the result of a contra-coup type of injury which is caused by the head striking an immovable object, such as a ringpost, a metal object or the floor," Dr. Larson explained. "When the object is resilient and movable, head injuries and contra-coup subarachnoid hemorrhages seldom occur. I know of no instance where death occurred from a punch on the head if the head was movable. A straight punch to the head while the head is in motion is incapable of causing serious injury or subarachnoid hemmorrhage because the contra-coup tearing of blood vessels does not occur unless the head is up against an immovable object."

During some 35 years of medical research on the subject, Dr. Larson read a great many articles regarding so-called "punch drunk" fistfighters.

"In my opinion," he told me, "the term 'punch drunk' is a misnomer. I don't think I have ever really seen individuals, who have gone into professional boxing with *normal* intelligence, wind up as so-called 'punch drunk' replicas of their former selves. Most prizefighters who were classified as such really had only low-level intelligence to begin with. Boxing had little to do with their mental deterioration. This is not to say, of course, that boxers have not received injuries which produced neurological symptoms, because history is saturated with such examples."

One of Dr. Larson's favorite "punch drunk" stories is about Lou Nova, another old heavyweight. It concerns the time Lou was sitting at ringside at a fight in California. A man came up to him with a small boy and said: "Lou, why didn't you show up at the house for dinner the other night?"

Dr. Larson picks up the rest of the story:

"Well, Lou looked at the man and knew he'd never seen him before, but he got the pitch right away. Sure, the man wanted to make a big impression on his son, and Lou had once fought the great Joe Louis for the heavyweight championship of the world. So Lou said: 'Oh, yes, I'm sorry. I wasn't able to make it. But the next time you invite me, I'll be there for sure.' Lou then turned to the little boy. 'So this is the little fellow you were telling me about?' The man said yes, that was his son. 'He's a fine, strapping boy,' Lou said. 'Now you take care of yourself, sonny, and some day you'll be a great football player or even a heavyweight champion.' Then the father said, 'Well, so long, Lou. Go ahead and watch the fight and I'll see you later.' 'Right,' Lou said, and as he turned away he heard the man speak to the boy. 'See?' the man was saying, 'didn't I tell you he was *punch drunk?*'"

Charles P. Larson was 17 years old when he signed up at Gonzaga in 1927. It was the Horatio Alger time of luck and pluck, rags and riches. So much to be seen and heard and learned in this America of adventurous growth!

When he was a junior, taking prelaw, for some reason related to balancing his school credits, he attended an evening class in bacteriology given by Dr. Robert F.E. Stier. Dr. Stier performed most of the autopsies for the coroner in the City of Spokane and throughout Spokane

County, as well as in some of the adjacent counties of eastern Washington.

Dr. Stier was a magnetic man with a natural zest for his work. He swept young Larson into the net of his enthusiasm, and Larson switched to premed with the idea from the beginning of specializing in forensic pathology—even before he selected his medical school.

As an undergraduate he worked with Dr. Stier, assisting him at many autopsies. Meanwhile, he managed to put away $10,000, every cent of which he earned himself, to defray his medical school costs. He was a fully matriculated, full-time student at Gonzaga all of that time. And as he is emphatic in pointing out, "I missed damned few of the dances."

Young Mr. Larson was on his own by this time. His father, the banker, faced adversity in the financial crash of '29, and the Farmers and Mechanics Bank failed. Larson, Sr. almost impoverished himself paying off all of his obligations. Then he and Mrs. Larson moved to River Falls, Wisconsin and started another bank, leaving son Charles behind to finish school at Gonzaga. Since then, some 50 years ago, he has been on his own, supporting himself, shaping his own destiny. That destiny has included seven children, all college graduates. Three sons have followed their father into medicine, while a fourth went into the practice of law.

While at Gonzaga, Larson acquired his first surgical instrument. On a visit to Jantzen Beach Amusement Park, in Portland, he was attracted to a "digger"—a glass box full of junky prizes which you tried to lever out in the jaws of a miniature crane by manipulating the handles on the outside. A nickel a try and you seldom got *anything*; especially you *never* got the "come-on" prize, which in this particular "digger" was a hunting knife that looked like a good one.

"That damn knife cost me pretty close to $15 in nickels before I finally snared it," Dr. Larson remembers. "But it was well worth it. It was a beauty. A Swedish knife with a magnificent steel blade, which I used for 10 years in performing autopsies and still keep as a memento. I have used it on probably 5,000 autopsies, including more than 1,000 I performed as the first Allied Army Medical Officer to go into Dachau, the Nazi concentration camp."

From Gonzaga, Larson went on to Medical School at McGill University in Montreal, where on his first day he walked in on Dr. Horst Oertel, one of the world's most celebrated pathologists. A crusty bachelor, Dr. Oertel was completely wedded to his work as Professor of Pathology and consultant in forensic pathology to the Canadian Pacific Railway.

"I walked into Dr. Oertel's office with all the confidence of youth," Dr. Larson recollected. "When he looked up, I said, 'I intend to be a forensic pathologist myself and I am ready to go to work for you as soon as I settle in.' He stared at me icily over his spectacles. He looked me up and down as if I were a disappointing laboratory specimen, started to say something that ended not in words, but in a weakened snort of indignation; weakened by my affrontery and his own shock over it."

The young medical student from Spokane found out later that almost everyone at McGill was scared to death of the elderly German, but Charley must have backed Professor Oertel's sails completely, for he put him to work the next day.

It should be put down right here that Charley Larson was out of character, or else his youth and enthusiasm got away from him that day; for Dr. Larson is a quiet, pleasantly mannered man, a *gentle* man with a quick smile that carries confidence and assurance in its warmth. Like most of the very *great* men of the world, he is simple in his tastes and very easy to approach. He builds no hard-to-climb outer fences about himself.

While he was a medical student at McGill and in constant need of funds, young Larson sold the Montreal *Herald* on the idea that he was a circulation hotshot from the States and set up for the paper a home-delivery network. The *Herald* never knew he was a would-be M.D. In a very short time he doubled the paper's circulation, whereupon he was fired because on a commission basis he was making in excess of $1,000 a month, which was more than the circulation manager got. That was enough to finish college.

At McGill, Larson learned fast enough to qualify during a pair of Christmas holiday periods as a volunteer assistant to Dr. Charles Norris, who was New York City's first chief medical examiner and a pioneer in the field. By his final year at McGill, he was a part-time but bread-winning pathologist at a Montreal hospital.

After completing his internship, young Larson—now *Doctor* Larson—went on to the University of Michigan and then to University of Oregon for a residency of special training.

The medical career of Dr. Charles P. Larson was on its way. Specialty: the science of pathology.

"There are three main divisions of the science of pathology," Dr. Larson explains. "Pathologic anatomy is one. That's the diagnosis of disease in the laboratory from tissues removed from the body. The anatomic pathologist is the man who goes into the operating room several times a day to stand by the operating surgeon to receive small pieces of tissue that have been excised, or to suggest to the surgeon what areas to go into for additional tissue that might facilitate diagnosis. He is the specialist who makes all the diagnoses from tissue examination.

"The second basic division of the science is clinical pathology. Clinical pathologists are doctors' doctors. They are highly specialized laboratory diagnosticians working in a very wide, very complicated and most sophisticated field of medical practice. The Pathology Laboratory at Tacoma General Hospital is equipped with a half-dozen machines and the service they perform is priceless, for when they establish the profile of a patient, the resulting diagnosis may be apparent.

"One of the subspecialties of clinical pathology is the *prevention* of disease. By running a complete laboratory profile on young, relative well people, the clinical pathologist may ascertain tendencies toward and *predict* arteriosclerosis, coronary disorder, diabetes, cancer and many of the other disorders of the body. Constraining the patient's conduct to suitable disciplines in his future living, plotting diets and supplementing diets can forestall or at least *postpone* what would have happened to him had sophisticated clinical pathology not intervened. To such an extent, the clinical pathologist can, in effect, become God's right hand—if longevity for all of us is God's will.

"The third division of the science is, of course, forensic pathology. The practice of forensic pathology is by no means limited to people who have ceased to be alive. It covers attempts at poisoning, the physical abuse of children, assaults and batteries, product liability and, of course, the entire field of medical and surgical malpractice. Medical malpractice suits are on a distinct upcurve, to such an extent at present that the premiums on malpractice insurance are so astronomical as to cause extreme hardship to young doctors. I have testified in several malpractice suits, and in spite of the tradition that physicians will not testify against each other, I have found the truth when I could. I have told the truth on the stand, and where I could, I have seen justice done regardless of its result on the medical careers involved.

"In the practice of forensic pathology as it pertains to criminal acts, it is most important that one comes on the scene *first*, before any ineptness smudges the picture. Called in time, I have the police authorities seal off the scene until I can get there. The state patrol sealed off 30 miles of freeway for me once, backing up several thousand cars on both sides of a body with a bullet hole in it—in a somewhat over-zealous compliance with my request. I firmly believe that if competent investigators reach the scene before it is distorted by slipshod procedure, *no one can get away with murder."*

Lady of the Lake

IT is said by the professionals that in every homicide there is one point in the investigation which is the key to the solution. But as carefully trained as a man may be—and as broadly experienced in his job—the very obviousness of that point can trip him. He comes up on it a dozen times and passes it by. In some subconscious way, it is possible that he may even blind himself to it, because of some unknown inhibition in his own makeup. That is why the work is often done in teams—that is why outside help is called in with the hope of turning up a new angle; that is why the CIA developed the formula of "in every step, follow a pattern of logic that is acceptable to more than one person."

Thereby hangs a true tale.

In 1939 Dr. Larson was given an innocent-looking length of rope. The rope, when followed to its beginning, led to the bottom of Crescent Lake, more than 5,000 feet deep in the lushly forested Olympic Mountains. The upper horn of the crescent that gives the lake its name is 18 miles from the waters of the Strait of Juan de Fuca, which separates the U.S. from Canada. At the bottom of the lake an underground stream flows three miles and empties, still underground, into Sullivan Lake. The Clallam Indians, aboriginal to the surrounding country, once believed that Crescent Lake was inhabited by demons—spirits which seized anyone who fell into the water—and *held* them under forever. Strangely, the nonmythical fact is, up to the time I'm writing about, the lake never *had* yielded the body of a victim of drowning. There were no "floaters." If a body went down, it stayed down.

Today the glassy mountain waters are endlessly furrowed by the oars of fishermen who don't know about evil spirits but are sure of trout and landlocked salmon.

One morning in the summer of 1939 the lake silence was broken acutely by two fishermen in a rowboat. They had snagged their hooks on an object which one of them thought was a woman's body—a bundle about five-and-a-half feet long, blanket-wrapped and roped with a foot sticking out and a white shoulder visible through a hole in the blanket. The other fisherman insisted it wasn't a human body at all. "It's more like a show-window dummy," he said. "A *manikin.*" It was not bloated as a human body would have been had it been submerged until abdominal gases gave it the necessary buoyancy to bring it to the surface. Nor was there an odor of decomposition, and the body, or effigy, only weighed 47 pounds.

Turned over to the local authorities, it was discovered to be the remains of a woman in her early 30s, but the mysteries of its weight, its nonbloat, its obvious failure to decompose were not solved. In the matter of identification, the auburn hair would be of help, but not the face, for, by water action or battering, it had become dehumanized to an extent that it was barely recognizable as a face.

An Oregon criminologist, Dr. Joseph Beeman, was called to the scene. Dr. Beeman agreed that it was a woman's body all right. Crescent's deep-freeze had remarkably preserved the body, and apparently the lake also contained an ample supply of the bacillus *aerobacter cloacae*, the organism that causes the slime on meat which spoils in water. Between the cold and the bacillus, a sort of chemical gear-shifting called *saponifaction* had taken place, turning the body almost completely to soap. The press was quick to give the mysterious dead woman a name: "The Lady of the Lake."

What the sheriff had was a poser even stickier than a whodunit—a who-is-it? For a long time, they still didn't know. Finally, Dr. Beeman, who had been chopping away at the enigma off and on, asked Dr. Larson to come in on the case.

To help him, Dr. Larson had five meager leads. He had a few strands of a woman's hair, which hadn't saponified, a bit of clothing and a scrap of her hose. He had the rope. And he had a six-tooth upper partial dental plate, which, if traced to the people who had made it, *could* identify the woman. Also, on the neck there were what were conceded to be ante-mortem (before death) bruises. Opposed bruises that thumb and fingers might have made by the act of strangling.

Under Dr. Larson's autopsy all of the interior organs turned out to be saponified, so that in effect, the Lady of the Lake was a five-and-a-half-foot, 47-pound bar of soap. And, yes, death had been brought about by strangulation, because in support of the evidence of the bruises on the neck, autopsy found the heart congested and the tissues of the neck showing evidence of old hemoglobin—positive indications of death by strangulation.

It was an acceptable conclusion that the body had originally been at such an extreme depth that there were no flesh-eating fish to destroy it. To support this conclusion, the rope that had secured the blanket around the body had a long loose end which was frayed into a "horse's tail," indicating that it had broken strand by strand from, quite possibly, a weight that had initially held the body on the lake's bottom.

Dr. Larson took water samples from the lake thousands of feet down and found the water to contain calcium and alkali, which with animal fat make soap. He also found that the waters on the bottom remained at approximately three degrees above freezing, which is the preservative temperature usually maintained in refrigerators.

He positioned the body initially in the backwash of the underground stream that flows from Crescent Lake into Sullivan Lake, thus accounting for the rapidity of saponification.

Dr. Larson goes on:

"Crescent Lake is a very deep lake; in fact, so deep in some places that it's hard to find the bottom. It's well over a mile deep in many places. It's a big lake and lots of people have drowned in it because of the sudden storms that come up.

"I will never forget looking at the Lady of the Lake for the first time. I'd never seen anything like it, but I'd read about things like it. Here was a body that had turned completely to soap. This is called adipocere formation, in which all the tissues of the body turn to soap. When they turn to soap, it's like that soap they advertise—it floats. I examined the body and made a few little incisions in the skin. I found nothing but soap. I'd take off a piece of it and put it in water, and it would float. Damnedest thing. I asked myself why the body hadn't decomposed; why did it turn to soap? I went up to Lake Crescent and took water samples. I had to go down in some places over a mile, letting out over 5,000 feet of line with a heavy lead weight on the end counterpoised to pull the lid off the bottle to get water samples. I cultured the bacterial content of the lake to determine what it was and whether there was anything there that would decompose a body. There were lots of organisms at that depth, but none would ferment or produce gas to bloat and decompose a body.

"Adipocere formation is not the result of bacteria, but the result of chemical transformation of the tissues of the body over a long period of time. You make soap out of animal fat, calcium and alkali, and the water was alkaline at this dept, and there is calcium in all water.

"What had happened was a chemical change in the body—it may take several years for this to happen—in which all the tissues turned to soap. The internal organs were all intact. We slowly came to the conclusion that this woman had been strangled because we found hemorrhages, the evidence of old hemoglobin in the tissues—the soap—of the neck—and those ante-mortem bruises. I then did a complete autopsy on her and determined she had not died of any natural causes. All of the organs were present and intact.

"This lead to a long chase. We still didn't know who this body had belonged to. We *did* know that we had a body of a woman who had been in the lake for several years, but the natives told us that of all the white people who had ever drowned there, not a one of them had ever returned to the surface. The Indians also had this in their ancient folklore. They were even afraid to fish the lake because, according to legend, there were evil spirits in the water. Indians who had drowned were lost forever.

"By soundings I found that underground stream which flows from Lake Crescent to Lake Sullivan. I got my sounding equipment down there (it was too deep for divers) and it stuck underneath a ledge where the current carried it into the stream. If you could ever get down underneath that ledge, you would probably find from 50 to 100 bodies, all of which have turned to soap. The water temperature at 5,000 feet didn't vary more than half a degree, summer to winter; the temperature of the water at that depth was around three degrees above freezing, the optimum temperature for adipocere formation. If the murderer of this woman had known these things, he'd never have bothered to weight her down; he'd have just thrown her into the lake and she'd never have been heard from again. Those are the mistakes killers make! That is what my job is really all about—finding those mistakes."

While Dr. Larson went about doing his thing, Hollis B. Fultz, a consulting criminologist from Olympia, beat the backwoods for clues trying to find out who the Lady of the Lake really was.

"Hollis was one of the best investigative detectives I've ever known," Dr. Larson said. "We worked on many cases together. But none more satisfying than Lady of the Lake."

One hunch Fultz had was Hallie Illingworth. She was married to a beer company salesman. They had lived in Port Angeles, about 20 miles from Lake Crescent. Hallie had worked as a sometimes waitress. Then, one day, she didn't show up for work. She just disappeared. That was in 1932. Fultz wondered about that.

Hallie Illingworth was about 36 at the time. Five-foot-six, 135 pounds. Good-looking, with beautiful auburn hair. Her husband, Monty, was the jealous type. He also drank too much. When he got in the booze, he often punched her out. He was mean to her. She'd show up at work with black eyes.

Fultz thought about this. He started asking around. Edgar Thompson, secretary of the Culinary Alliance, where Hallie belonged to the local union, said she had not bothered to get a transfer card.

"If she left town voluntarily," he said, "I'd have thought she would have come and got a transfer card so she could get a job some place else. She was a good worker. She could work anywhere. You know," Edgar Thompson said, "if it wasn't for the fact she's been gone so long, I'd say she's the Lady of the Lake."

Edgar said, yes, there were relatives. She had a sister, Lois Latham, a member of the same union. But she'd moved to Fort Peck, Montana, he said. No, he didn't know what became of her after that.

At the request of Fultz, Thompson wrote to all the unions in Montana. Did anyone know the whereabouts of Lois Latham? There was no success.

In Fultz's search, he ran across Mrs. Nina Carlsen, a former close friend of Lois Latham. Mrs. Carlsen lived at Sequim, 19 miles southeast of Port Angeles. She said the last she heard from Lois she was married to a government guard and living at College Place, Washington—near Walla Walla.

The plot was thickening. Lois was located. She said she hadn't heard from her sister since Christmas, 1932. None of the family had heard from her.

"Hallie came to the apartment where I lived with Elinore Pearson, a stenographer, about the middle of the afternoon," Lois recalled. "She stayed till dinnertime, then went out when Elinore came home. Later, Monty showed up looking for Hallie. I told him she'd been there but had gone. The next morning he came into The Loop, the restaurant where I worked, and asked if I'd seen Hallie. The time was 6:30 a.m. No, I told him, I'd not seen her since yesterday at the apartment. He looked dreadful, like he'd slept in his clothes. He explained he'd been at an all-night beer bust at Port Townsend. He said he and Hallie had a big fight when he got home and he stormed out. His eyes were bleary and he looked like he was going to cry. I didn't see Monty for 24 hours. The next day he came to the apartment and asked if I'd seen Hallie. I told him no. He shook his head, sadly. Some Christmas, he said, and walked out. There were tears in his eyes.

"I didn't see Monty again for a week. When he did show up, finally, he said he hadn't told me everything. 'Hallie's left me,' he said. 'After our big fight, she packed a suitcase and said she was never coming back,' he said. 'She said none of us would ever see her again. I think she's gone to that Navy Lt. Commander fella down at Bremerton. I never did trust him.' Hallie had known this Navy officer since 1931. Monty was always jealous of him."

Lois was asked if she had heard from Monty lately.

"Only through Elinore Pearson," Lois said. "She writes regularly. She and Monty are married now and living in Long Beach, California. She often asks if I ever hear from Hallie."

The trail was growing hotter. Fultz could smell blood. He next talked to Mrs. James Johnson of Vancouver, Washington. She was another of Hallie's sisters. Mrs. Johnson studied the photos of the Lady of the Lake that Fultz handed her, and said, "That's Hallie's form, all right. And she had high cheekbones like the photos show. Her hair was exactly the color of this and she had a partial upper plate."

After leaving Mrs. Johnson, Fultz drove up to Lake Pleasant, 50 miles from Port Angeles, and talked to Jessie Hudson, an old friend of Hallie's who ran a cookhouse for a mill crew there. She was well-known for her photographic memory.

"Hallie had a partial upper plate," Jessie said, "but I never saw it. Once, at the restaurant where we worked the same shift, she walked in with black and blue marks on her throat; she often did. 'Monty and I had another fight,' she said. 'He nearly strangled me to death. He'll kill me some day. Last night, he broke a tooth out when he hit me.' I asked her to show me the tooth and she said it was in a partial upper plate which she had left with the dentist for repair."

Fultz then showed her the photos. Her eyes filled with tears when she looked at them.

"Yes," she said, "that's her hair—and that's her body. And, yes, that's her dress. I sold it to her. I was working at J.C. Penney in 1932, and she walked in and bought that dress."

Jessie rubbed her chin, thoughtfully.

"Say," she said, "do you notice anything peculiar about her right foot?"

"What's wrong with her right foot?" Fultz wanted to know.

"Well, look at it," Jessie said. "See that big bunion? Hallie had a bunion so big she always kidded the salesman, saying she wanted a one size larger shoe for that foot. Yes, sir, that's Hallie's foot, all right."

That settled it. Hollis Fultz was convinced. Hallie Illingworth was the Lady of the Lake.

The Lady of the Lake was wearing a green wool dress that still carried J.C. Penney's label. The style of the dress dated it at about 10 years before the body surfaced. The nearest J.C. Penney store was in Port Angeles. There the dress was identified as stock the store had carried approximately 10 years before, but no records of individual names or purchasers had been kept.

On the body were *rayon*, not silk or cotton, stockings. Rayon being wartime stocking material, this fact added confirmation to the dating profile that Dr. Larson was drawing. He had cuttings from the stocking analyzed in the laboratory at the University of Puget Sound, for there was a period in the process of manufacturing rayon when lead was used as a filler.

When you burn a piece of rayon stocking of that vintage, you can see little bubbles of lead in the crumbly ash of the fibre. Those tiny bubbles were evident, and this further bracketed the time limit to approximately the same 10 years of the dress. So Dr. Larson and his ace gumshoe, Hollis Fultz, were now back-trailing a woman who had been missing for nearly 10 years from *somewhere.* Port Angeles? Hallie Illingworth? Fultz was betting on Hallie, but they still had to be sure.

All leads were tracked down. For example, a complete chart of The Lady's dental work had been made and circularized in professional dental journals from coast to coast. Drs. Larson and Beeman became steady if modest advertisers. For months, they ran ads picturing the bridgework, in the hope that the dentist who made it would recognize the partial plate.

It was some 20 months before a reply came, because the dentist who finally responded, Dr. A.J. McDowell of Foulkton, South Dakota, did not read his journals regularly, but let them go for long periods and then caught up by a concentrated spate of intensive reading. He stated that he had made a partial upper denture like the one advertised—for a Hallie Spraker—13 years before. He further stated that Hallie Spraker (Spraker was the name of her first husband) had no molars whatever in her lower jaw. Nor did the saponified body.

"Mrs. Spraker later moved to Port Angeles," Dr. McDowell wrote in his letter. The body now had a name and an approximate date of death by strangulation.

Dr. McDowell thus made life much less confusing for the doctor-detectives. Many people in Port Angeles remembered Hallie. She had married a beer salesman named Monty Illingworth. In 1932, she had run off to Alaska with a sailor, they said, or so her husband had told them. Shortly thereafter Monty had departed for California in the company of a town charmer. There were even several residents who thought they had seen Hallie on the streets of Fairbanks, which just goes to show that you can't believe everything people tell you.

And then there was the rope—the rope that had tied the blanket around Hallie. It was a three-strand, half-inch rope that had an identifying blue fibre of about the thickness of a hair running through the center strand. A description of this rope was circularized to manufacturers all over the U.S. and Canada, and information eventually came back to the effect that Sears, Roebuck in Port Angeles was the only outlet in the area that sold that particular brand.

Among sales of record at Sears, one thousand feet of this rope was sold to a resort owner on Crescent Lake for tying up his rental boats. Dr. Larson personally talked with the fellow and was satisfied he had nothing to do with the murder.

Dr. Larson was about to leave when the boathouse man suddenly remembered lending a hundred feet of the rope to a beer salesman one time when his truck got mired in some mud. He remembered the loan because the rope was not returned or ever paid for. That, oddly enough, was how the dentist in South Dakota remembered Hallie Spraker. She had left town without paying him.

All beer salesmen in the area at the time were traced until a "possible" was found. It turned out to be Monty Illingworth, who had, at one time, a somewhat plump wife, with auburn hair and the first name of Hallie. His wife was remembered to have bought her clothing at J.C. Penney and she had once been married to a man named Spraker.

All the coins now fell into the slot. Illingworth was extradited from California and indicted. He said that his wife had gone off to Alaska with another man, but the jury did not buy the sketchy supporting evidence Monty offered.

Dr. Larson took the stand and with great enthusiasm put on a demonstration that is still talked about in the Pacific Northwest by those who saw it. In a saucer he burned pieces of rayon, silk and cotton stockings to differentiate the odor and ash of one from the others and to show the jury the tiny lead bubbles in the stockings found on Hallie Illingworth's body, thus dating her death, because rayon stockings first came on the Port Angeles market in 1931. He then asked for a glass of water into which he dropped a small piece of saponified tissue which he had excised from the body. It went straight to the bottom of the glass then slowly rose to the top as Hallie's saponified body had done after the frayed rope released the weight that had originally held it to the bottom of Crescent Lake.

It took the jury less than an hour to find Monty Illingworth guilty of murder in the second degree. He was sentenced to life imprisonment in the Washington State Penitentiary at Walla Walla.

Postscript:

While researching the Lady in the Lake, I talked to two members of the cast, Hollis Fultz and Mrs. John Bayton of Port Angeles. At the time of the investigation, Mrs. Bayton worked in the Clallam County Sheriff's Department. She served as the bailiff during the trial of Monty Illingworth. Mrs. Bayton was 90 when I visited her, and she remembered the case as though it were the day before yesterday.

"I remember when Hallie's body was brought to Port Angeles," she said. "I remember when I touched it, it felt just like soap. An eerie sensation. When the sheriff opened up the blankets that were roped around it, there was an almost perfectly formed woman—from the shoulders down. The face, of course, from years of submersion, was unrecognizable, but there was her partial upper dental plate still in place. I didn't know it then, but it was to turn out, after Dr. Larson came on the case, that I knew that dead woman as well as I knew members of my own family."

Mrs. Bayton remembered that the trial lasted for nine days. The courtroom was jammed to overflowing. Newsmen from all over the country came to cover the case of the Lady of the Lake. Mrs. Bayton saw Hallie's sister at the trial and went over and put some loose coins in her hand.

"What's this?" she wanted to know.

Mrs. Bayton told her, "I took them out of Hallie's pocket when her body was brought in."

There must have been $5 in change.

The last tips Hallie ever got.

Hollis Fultz was an amazing man. He was not a doctor or a policeman. He was a special investigator. He had the same two-and-two-makes-four approach to the details of a crime as Dr. Larson does to a dead body.

Fultz started life as a newspaper man. From general reporting he began to be assigned to the police beat. But long before that, when a crime was in the papers, he would mull the details over and usually come up with something. He would go to the police, and almost invariably, if they acted on his suggestion, they'd hit pay dirt.

One night, several years ago, Dr. Larson and I paid Fultz a visit. He was then 88 and still serving, unopposed, as coroner of the City of Olympia. Inevitably, the conversation got around to murders and how to solve them.

"If you can tell me the exact time at which someone has been murdered, I believe I can tell you who killed him," Hollis said. "No mystery. You start checking out all of the people who were the victim's close friends and ask them where they were at the time. Sooner or later one of them will start lying to you. Check out the lies for truth and you will, nine times out of 10, have the murderer. It's a sad fact, but true, that usually one of a man's friends murders him, because only a fool lets his enemies get close enough."

Hollis chuckled. "And if you want the exact time of death," he added, "Dr. Larson can come as close as anybody."

"Add to that," Dr. Larson said, "if a man commits any crime—that if he's at the scene long enough and the scene is investigated by experts—invariably they will turn up some evidence that he has been there. It is impossible for a man not to leave some evidence behind if he has stopped in any one place long enough. By long enough, let's say two minutes—or three."

"There isn't any such thing as a perfect crime, because if you even suspect there *has* been a crime, it is not perfect," Fultz said. "What we are faced with in most cases is imperfectly trained homicide investigators and poorly qualified medical examiners. Medical examiners should, by law, be required to be specialized forensic pathologists—and a good forensic pathologist ought to be more than half-cop!"

"Like Dr. Larson?" I asked.

"Like Dr. Larson," Fultz answered.

War Is Hell

WITH an M.D. from McGill, Dr. Larson went on to the University of Michigan and University of Oregon for further study. For two years, he taught at UO as a lecturer in pathology and in *neuropathology*, the study of the causes of disease and malfunction of the human nervous system. He then spent a short time in additional study at the Mayo Clinic. He also took courses in ballistics and firearm identification and document examination from the experts at the Chicago Police Department. Against that background he was appointed pathologist to the Tacoma General Hospital in 1938.

Like millions of other Americans, life went along against a background of sad expectancy all around. A lot of them only walked through the motions. Living was like watching a film they had every reason to believe was new, only to realize they had seen it all before.

In Europe the last surviving dynasties were falling, nations collapsing, politics changing and dictators ranting. Once more the armies of traditional enemies were marching side by side as allies toward the inevitability of another world war. Germany had started to gobble up Austria and Czechoslovakia; the day was not far off when she would join with Soviet Russia, who had already swept across the tiny Baltic countries of Estonia, Latvia and Lithuania, to devour Poland.

Along the western redoubt of the European continent, Belgium, the Netherlands and Denmark braced for the holocaust that was yet to come, while a self-deluded France huddled behind the Maginot Line.

On Saturday morning at one o'clock, October 1, 1938, the Munich crisis reached its climax when 600 gray-clad German soldiers crossed the border to begin the occupation of Czechoslovakia. In a few stunned hours the world came to the realization that war was not only threatening but imminent. Here in the United States, the knowledge was forcibly borne home that the nation's detachment from world affairs had ended. For a lot of college athletes the drama of the day came down to an even finer point of tension. Many of them that afternoon were in football uniforms on campus playing fields, and the world passed from one period to another almost between the opening kickoff and the final whistle of their games.

In 1941, immediately after Pearl Harbor, Dr. Larson volunteered and was given a reserve commission in the Medical Corps, Army of the United States. After a stultifying base hospital routine of prostatic massage and paint-them-with-iodine-and-mark-them-duty, he hit Omaha Beach in Normandy with the advance party of the 50th General Army Hospital. This unit was set up under canvas at Carentan, where it stayed until Paris was taken. It then moved into the Verdun area.

While Dr. Larson was at Verdun, that mysterious machine in the subcellars of the Pentagon was programmed to find forensic pathologists. When the wheels stopped whirring, it came up with the only two that were serving at that time in the European Theatre. Major Charles P. Larson, 35, and Dr. Vincent Sneedon, who today is Professor of Pathology at the University of Oregon.

"Dr. Sneedon was not primarily a *forensic* pathologist," Dr. Larson told me recently, "so I believe I was the only forensic pathologist on duty in the entire European Theater—which is why I was detailed ultimately to conduct the autopsies at Dachau. So whether the authorities liked what I did or not, they were stuck with the only top-qualified man in my field and they had to take me!"

Major Larson was thus assigned to the Judge Advocate General's Department, which detail made him a combatant soldier. He took off his Red Cross armband, drew a duty belt and holster and stuffed a .45 caliber equalizer into it.

Ordered into Paris, he was interviewed, briefed and then detailed to War Crime's Investigation Team Number 6823, covering all of south Germany, under the command of Colonel David Chavez of the distinguished New Mexico family. The mission of the team from initially investigating war crimes only against American personnel was broadened to include German war crimes against all humanity.

Part of the team made its temporary headquarters in Seeshaupt, near Munich. About two days before Major Larson arrived, Allied bombers had had a field day with key targets in and around the town, and during the raid a freight train full of concentration camp prisoners was strafed. "Some were shot by German machine guns as the easiest way to keep them from escaping in the confusion," Dr. Larson recalled.

When Major Larson arrived, all of the prisoners were dead in the cars. He took pictures with an old 35 mm Kodak of the evidence showing the dead crammed together like cattle. He autopsied a representative sample to indicate that while some had died from shots from above during the strafing runs of the plane, most had been done to death by machine gun fire from both sides of the track.

Major Larson's official report of the atrocity follows:

5 May, 1945—Seeshaupt Incident—Pathologist Report:

On 3 May, 1945, at 1400 hours, I inspected a German train at the above location. This portion of the train consisted of approximately 60 boxcars and flatcars in which approximately 1,500 prisoners and slave-laborers of all nationalities were being transported to another location in Germany on 26 April, 1945.

65 dead bodies were found in various boxcars of the train. 38 of these were men who had been killed by gunshot wounds and 3 were women who died in the same fashion; 24 bodies showed no cause of death from external examination. All of these bodies were in a most pitiful condition, being clothed in rags, the majority having no shoes and insufficient blankets. There were no sanitary facilities aboard the train and the flatcars had no tops, leaving the occupants of these cars exposed to the elements. The flat-tops were covered with barbed wire which left a space only 3 feet high for those occupying these cars. All of the bodies inspected were emaciated, infested with lice and had apparently been dead for about a week. A few of the bodies in which no known cause of death was observed had an *erthyematous* (red) rash which could have been due to typhus. Practically all of the bodies were filthy dirty, indicating that the people had had no opportunity to bathe for a long time. Most of the bodies had either decubitus sores and/or infected wounds and ulcers of a minor character on various parts of the body. Personal effects were practically nil, but identification was possible by means of numbers tatooed on arms and chests. Of those who had been shot many had not died immediately, as there was evidence of attempts at first aid treatment by means of paper dressings. The majority appeared to have been shot by .50 cal. machine-gun ammunition, but others showed evidence of having been killed by small-arms fire. A .50 cal. machine gun bullet was recovered, but no small arms bullets were found in the examination, as most of them had passed entirely through

the bodies. Many of the flatcars showed evidence of having been strafed from the air.

On 5 May, 1945, I inspected the Seeshaupt German Military Luftwaffe Hospital which was caring for the injured and ill moved from the train. From all appearances they were receiving excellent care. There were 163 patients in the hospital, 35 of whom had been injured by gun fire. The balance were composed of those suffering from severe malnutrition, tuberculosis and typhus fever; 9 patients had died since the patients were first received. In questioning the German military doctors who had performed the surgery on the surgical cases, they stated that the majority of their cases had been injured by large caliber ammunition, but that there were some who appeared to have been injured by small arms fire. The projectiles which had been removed by surgery had been given back to the patients as souvenirs.

2. STALTART INCIDENT:

This small village is located approximately 6 km due south of Seeshaupt, and on the railroad siding there were about 40 flat-tops and boxcars similar to those described in the first incident. In fact this was part of the same train which had been dropped off before reaching Seeshaupt; 17 bodies were found in the cars of this portion of the train, 16 of which showed no external cause of death. The condition of these bodies was the same as that described in the first incident. One body had been shot in the head by small arms fire in two places and also through the right chest. Witnesses stated that this man had been murdered by an SS soldier 10 minutes before the Americans arrived in town.

One woman was included among the 17 bodies found at this location.

SIGNED: Charles P. Larson, Major M.C.
Pathologist-War Crimes Team 6823
0477636.

Whereas Dr. Larson over 40 years has become inured to the fact of death—even to the fact of violent death—he still finds himself strangely reluctant to open up the subject of the German concentration camps, of the ghastly crematoriums and the atrocious medical experimentation on helpless humanity—the brutality, the out-and-out sadism, the cold-blooded academic heartlessness.

"I imagine that this is because I must have a latent feeling of shock over the whole frightful business," he told me in 1978. "*That* I will carry to my grave. I can live with it as long as it is dormant, but I hate to bring it back now into remembered fact."

However, most heavily-shot-over combat veterans have that same reluctance. The rule is that, win or lose, *never* revisit an old battlefield. The memory of warfare is only tolerable because of the outrageously humorous incidents that bubble up through the primeval slime.

In the Seeshaupt area Major Larson's team was billeted in the palatial home of the Baron Rudolph von Simolon who had owned the Mercedes-Benz plant at Stuttgart. The von Simolon family was still in shock when the Americans arrived, for when they took the town, the Baron had shot himself. He was a polio cripple and a friend apparently of Franklin D. Roosevelt, for his study wall was covered with pictures of the two of them together.

The bereaved hausfrau asked Major Larson to look in on her 22-year-old daughter who was suffering from a leg infection. He found the young woman in agonizing pain and running an alarming temperature. In the way you learn to do things in wartime, he sent his driver out to liberate some penicillin. The driver was so successful so quickly that Major Larson was shortly able to give the girl 10,000 units which cured the infection, lowered the temperature and saved her life. Nor did her mother, the hausfrau, have any doubt that the American doctor had saved her daughter, for she told him that he might have anything of theirs he wanted for his fee. Major Larson explained to the mother that he was no longer in private practice and that she might therefore consider his services as a by-product of the American war effort.

In spite of his ineptness with the German language,

Major Larson realized very shortly that Hausfrau Simolon was very much embarrassed by lack of money, and that she was construing his refusal of a fee as an act of charity. When she continued to press him to accept some tangible gift of gratefulness, he did.

In extenuation of what he did, in order that it may not be misconstrued, today he will put forth the defense that a man is only young once and that war is war, so that when she offered it to him, he took the late Baron's 16 cylinder red Mercedes-Benz convertible coupe which was then valued at around $35,000.

Only three cars like that had ever been made. Hitler had one. Goering had one—and now Major Charles P. Larson, from Tacoma, Washington, USA, damned well had one. Hausfrau von Simolon made it official by signing the necessary papers over to him.

It was practically a new car, a beautiful maroon and a magnificent machine to drive. Very shortly thereafter, however, Major Larson made a tactical blunder. He parked it at Army Headquarters in Augsburg and an American general, who shall be nameless except for the names Major Larson called him under his breath, saw it. He wanted it. Very generously he authorized Major Larson to go to the motor pool and pick out any *other* car he fancied—but he held out his hand for the papers on the Major's Mercedes-Benz and said, "I will return it to Hausfrau von Simolon when I am finished with it."

The Major picked out a modest black Mercedes—valued at about $6,000—as a consolation prize. The general was killed in his 16-cylinder job a few weeks later when at top speed he failed to negotiate a turn on a mountain road. That story still hurts Dr. Larson to tell—for that machine was a beauty—and the general totaled it!

Prior to Seeshaupt, Major Larson's Investigation Team had been ordered to go to the Hammelsburg Camp, which contained only commissioned officer POWs. The armies were still moving, and the situations everywhere were dangerously fluid. It was rumored that General Patton was broadening one arm of his advance to include Hammelsburg in order to free his son-in-law. So Major Larson took his legal officer, Captain Walker, and his hard-bitten Pfc. Driver Bocock, who also acted as his interpreter. About an hour and a half out of Augsburg the road branched right and left. At the intersection there was a sign, "Hammelsburg," with an arrow, so they took that road, failing entirely to see a much smaller sign, "Hammelsburg Camp," on the other road.

A few minutes later they rolled into the town square of Hammelsburg, a pleasant little Christmas-card place of about 10,000 population, completely untouched by the grimy hands of war. There were a dozen or so German soldiers in uniform in the square, singly and in twos and threes, but they were totally indifferent to the Americans' presence. A dreadful inertia bears down upon combat soldiers and makes old men of them in very short time. Add to that the apathy of accepted defeat and you have men that have gone beyond human awareness. They look, but they do not see, nor do they care. They listen, but they do not hear. They eat, but they do not taste. They are alive, but they do not live. Such were the scattered German soldiers at Hammelsburg.

Major Larson told Pfc. Bocock to drive slowly around the square to what looked to be the City Hall. Shortly after they stopped, His Honor the Mayor came out, a white sheet in his hand, and surrendered the town to *Major Larson.* With that dozens of the townspeople converged upon the Americans waving napkins, shirts and pillow cases, confirming the fact that their mayor had spoken for them, and they were surrendering.

Under international law Major Larson was in a somewhat anomalous position. Captain Walker was not quite sure of the legal remifications of the matter. Nevertheless on the impulse of the moment, Major Larson accepted the surrender with a few impromptu—if not immortal—words which Bocock translated. Meanwhile, he kept a tommy-gun across his knees, the muzzle pointed toward the German soldiers in the square.

Having surrendered, the mayor said he wanted Major Larson to meet someone. He disappeared inside the City Hall and came back out a few minutes later with a chap who looked to be British. He had an engaging grin, dirty-blond, crew-cut hair, was medium size and about 30.

"Major," the mayor said, "meet the King of Hammelsburg."

A very personable chap, "The King." And a very privileged character. He was a corporal in the British Army. The Germans captured him early in the war, and he was sitting out the fighting at Hammelsburg Camp, except that he was seldom there. He came and went as he pleased between camp and town. He was married to a German woman and had three children. He also had a wife and children back in England.

"Everybody liked him," Dr. Larson remembers. "Congenial, highly trusted, he had a pass to leave Hammelsburg Camp anytime he wanted to go into town. Everybody called him the 'King of Hammelsburg.' So as King, he really took care of us. He had us occupy the City Hall, made of stone, and then instructed the good hausfraus of the community to bring us a fabulous home-cooked meal. That night, he invited me over to his house. There was still a lot of snipers' fire going on in the nearby woods, yet the King said, 'Come on, nothing will happen.' So I went off in the night with the King of Hammelsburg—right in the middle of a war. Hell, I *trusted* him as much as the Germans did. Through back alleys, along dark streets, we worked our way to the other side of town, where we finally entered a well-furnished house. I met his wife and children, and then we got down to the real business. He brought out a bottle of fine, ancient bourbon. We toasted the British—the Americans—ultimate victory. I got smashed. I don't even remember going back to City Hall. The King walked me back, and the next day he issued an order to have all firearms, and all other weapons in private possession, brought in and dumped in the square. He then had the stocks broken from the rifles and shotguns, the revolvers and auto pistols snapped short at the hilt. The lot was then burned. Watching those priceless antiques go up in smoke broke my heart, for I was a collector and some of those ancestral weapons brought in by the people of Hammelsburg were book pieces."

The Mayor of Hammelsburg then formally issued a proclamation (a copy of which hangs framed in Dr. Larson's study today), to the effect that he had surrendered his Town to Number 6218 War Crimes Team, Major Charles P. Larson, M.D., commanding.

"Then the King accompanied me out to Hammelsburg Camp," Dr. Larson recalls. "He was even respected out there. Everybody liked him. He was very popular, even though he had special privileges. Even the prisoners called him the King of Hammelsburg. Damn, what a guy. He was the most unique character I met in the war."

After Seeshaupt, Major Larson and his War Crimes Team investigated the Kauffring Camps. When they got there, Major Larson had an American autopsy assistant assigned to him by the Army. But after the assistant saw all the dead bodies, he quit. Major Larson got through to the highest military command and asked for assistance. Nobody wanted anything to do with it. But Major Larson was told of a German prison camp nearby where he might find some help. So the team drove over to the compound and talked to the American Army officer in charge. The officer called in a couple of English-speaking Germans, and the Germans broadcast Major Larson's call over the camp loudspeaker for volunteers with previous experience in performing autopsies. There were about 20,000 prisoners in the camp—but only one German volunteered. He was a college man from the southern part of Germany and was experienced.

Major Larson brought him in for an interview. He didn't speak English, but he did speak French. Major Larson had fair French but no German, so they talked in French.

"He's a bad risk," the Camp Commander warned Major Larson. "He's a hidebound Nazi and will cause you trouble."

The young man was in his late 20s, with typical Germanic features. He was strong and healthy, and fit for the work in hand.

Major Larson asked him, "If I take you, will you gun me in the back the first chance you get?"

He shook his head. "If you get me out of this *couseur* (sewer), I'll gun any man who tries to gun you in the back!" he said. His first name was Hans and he served as Major Larson's autopsy assistant for the next two months, including the work at Dachau.

At the first autopsy they did together, Major Larson handed Hans an enormous hunting knife and told him to get busy. The good doctor always used hunting knives in his autopsy work because they are easy to keep sharp. He used them for years, before he started using disposable blades on Bard-Parker handles. Major Larson brought his own hunting knives from the United States, with long handles and big blades. He gave Hans one and he handled it very skillfully. Together they performed three times as many autopsies as the doctor could have done alone. In fact, Hans was so good that Major Larson was able to turn him loose and let him do the autopsy while the Major wrote the notes. This was excellent. Their garbled French improved daily, and Hans even learned some English.

One of their first assignments at Kauffring was to investigate the mass graves. It was a suffocating experience. The Major had seen a lot of death in his time, but nothing like what he found in those block-long graves. There were 10,000 bodies lying out there in those death trenches.

After the first mass grave was uncovered by a bulldozer, Major Larson and Hans found there were at least ten more nearby where thousands more bodies had been buried—piled up six high like cordwood. Major Larson had to find out how all those poor people died.

There was no house, no place, to do a proper autopsy. This was in early May and the southern part of Germany, near the Alps, was still quite chilly and wet. Major Larson and Hans found some old lumber, built a table and set it alongside the first open grave. Then they brought up one of the bodies and started doing the autopsy. Major Larson was wearing his steel helmet because he didn't have any other hat and suddenly—ZING!—a bullet caromed off it. They'd been in the area for only 48 hours and American ground troops hadn't had time as yet to clear the surrounding woods of enemy snipers.

Major Larson yelled, "Let's get the hell out of here!" They jumped into their jeep and drove slam-bang until they came to an abandoned farmhouse below a distant knoll. The blinds were pulled. There was no sign of life. They walked in. The Major was ahead of Hans. At the front was a long corridor with two doors. One door led to a narrow living room, the other to the bedrooms. Major Larson chose the door to the left—and walked smack into a living room jammed full of Nazi soldiers. They were fully armed, dog dirty and loaded for bear. The instant Hans saw the Germans, he shouted, "Achtung!" and the room snapped to attention. Major Larson got his .45 out fast.

The Germans offered no resistance. Hans went around the room gathering up their weapons, and then he filed them out of the farmhouse and lined them up in front of the jeep. They were only about five kilometers from the prison camp where the Major had originally found Hans, so they marched their prisoners down the road to the camp. One shaken American Major behind the wheel of a jeep and 30 Nazi soldiers, hands over their heads, clumping on ahead of him! What a war!

Hans turned out to be quite a guy, and Major Larson's greatest worry was what was going to become of him after the work was done. Most captured Nazis were being sent to prison, and Major Larson didn't want to see that happen to Hans. He felt the young man deserved a break. Frankly, he seriously considered bringing him back to the States and setting him up in his Tacoma office as an assistant.

When their work together was finished, Major Larson gave Hans all the money he had, along with a personal letter explaining how much value he had been in the Major's work and how loyal and trustworthy Hans had been. Hans departed with this and that's the last Major Larson ever saw or heard of him. He gave Hans his home address back in Tacoma, but he never heard from him again. He believes Hans must have been killed somewhere down the line.

The first Kauffring Camps that Team Number 6823 investigated were located on the east side of the Rhine, situated in and around the town of Landsburg, Germany. There the team ran into a fairly large number of small prison camps where numerous atrocities had been committed. It must be pointed out that in all the prison camps Major Larson investigated there was one basic policy under the Germans: the prisoners were expected to work and produce materiel needed by the Army. The prisoners were all underfed and poorly housed. Barracks were deplorable. They all wore similar clothing and were unprotected against the winter weather. They were so closely packed together that sanitation was practically nonexistent, and consequently they suffered from multiple diseases. They were all very poorly nourished, but the German people, themselves, had very little to eat in the last year of the war. With food in such short supply, we can imagine how poorly fed the prisoners were. It was miraculous any of them lived as long as they did.

These, then, are Major Larson's original reports on the Kauffring Camps:

Subject: Investigation of atrocities at Kauffring Camp #4 near Hulach, Germany. (Hulach is near Landsburg).

On May 1, 1945, I inspected 286 bodies lying in the compound of the above camp. The examination as to the cause of death was of necessity quite superficial and hurried. The causes of death could be roughly divided into three categories:

1. 86 bodies were so severely burned that the burns themselves were undoubtedly the cause of death. Sworn statements of witnesses indicate that these individuals were locked in the barracks at the compound and that these buildings were deliberately set on fire with the attempt to destroy all these bodies by the Germans shortly before the American troops liberated this camp.

2. 11 bodies were shot either in the head, chest or abdomen or in different combinations of the above wounds sufficient to be the cause of death.

3. 189 bodies showed no gross external cause of death. All of these bodies, as well as those in the foregoing two classifications, were extremely emaciated; many of them had large decubitus sores, and all were lice-infested. According to witnesses, typhus was present in this camp and some of these could have died of this disease. However, according to other reliable testimony, these individuals were murdered by the hypodermic injection of an unknown poison a matter of hours before the Americans liberated the camp. The German doctor for the camp—a "Dr. Blanke"—was seen to have used a large syringe with a needle and to have injected this unknown poison into these individuals. The result of the injection was death in from five to 20 minutes. Death was preceeded by generalized convulsions. In a search of the camp and of "Dr. Blanke's" home and office, no clue was found as to the type of poison used. From some autopsies performed, the brain, portions of the liver, the spleen, the heart and one kidney were retained for transmission to the First Medical Laboratory in Paris for toxicological examination to determine the type of poison administered. (Author's Note: Major Larson later received reports from the FML in Paris that the organs he had sent in for toxicological examination on three autopsied cases were *negative* for all poisons.) In one autopsied case the

individual had pulmonary tuberculosis which was bilateral and rather far advanced. There was no gross cavitation, and about 75 percent of the lung tissue contained air and was not completely replaced by the tuberculosis except for some recent bronchogenic dissemination. No focal tuberculosis was found in other organs of the body. This autopsy was performed under field conditions with no water available.

The testimony suggested that some of those poisoned received the injection into the chest over the heart. No needle wounds were observed on the heart in the cases autopsied.

Dr. Blanke committed suicide a few minutes before the Americans arrived in town and, according to testimony, his death was due to poisoning self-administered, supposedly the same type used on the prisoners in the compound. He also murdered his wife by the same means before taking his own life.

Thirty-one additional bodies were found in the woods lying on the ground in a somewhat scattered position a few hundred yards from the compound. Superficial examination of these bodies showed that 17 of them had died as a result of gunshot wounds; mostly multiple and probably from machine gun fire as whole extremities were amputated on some. Fourteen of these bodies showed no visible external cause of death and were also supposed to have been poisoned. Numerous photographs were taken to corroborate this report.

SIGNED: Major C.P. Larson, M.C.
Pathologist (50th General Hospital)
D.S. with War Crimes Team 6823.

On the *west* side of the Rhine, the Kauffring Camps were in the same condition as what Major Larson had been hearing about Dachau, except that there was no evidence of medical experimentation on human beings. The prisoners had all been on war munitions work—and on starvation rations. The bodies were unbelievably emaciated. The stench was sickening. To counteract the smell,

Major Larson discovered long ago that by spreading Noxema inside his surgical mask, all he was conscious of was a pleasant, cool, mentholated fragrance.

When the Germans realized the Allies were near enough to liberate those camps, they machine-gunned some of the remaining prisoners. Mass graves were discovered about 10 kilometers from the camps. In one grave the bulldozers uncovered an estimated 2,000 bodies, many of which were subjected to autopsy examination by Major Larson. All of those autopsied had died of various conditions such as emaciation with starvation, tuberculosis, typhus or other infectious diseases. The entire living prison population of some camps had been liquidated in one brief quarter of an hour prior to the arrival of the Allied Armies.

Shortly after the fall of Munich, Major Larson went on to Dachau with his war crimes investigating team. Dachau was located about 10 kilometers from Munich.

This most horrible of prisons was sealed up tight as a drum. Inside an American Engineer battalion had gotten hold of some DDT and was spraying everybody because a typhus epidemic was spreading like wildfire. Typhus spreads from one person to another by infected lice, and all the dead were crawling with lice.

This was in June, 1945. Dr. Larson remembers the date well, because it was just about that time the papers came down from high command that he had been promoted to Lt. Colonel. He was now going to earn the extra pay.

To get into Dachau, you had to have a pass. Col. Larson's was signed by the Commanding General of the area. (He still has the original.) For the next 10 days, many nights with only an hour or two of restless sleep, Col. Larson worked among the dead. He performed about 25 autopsies a day and superficially examined another 300 to 1,000 bodies. He autopsied only those bodies that appeared to have died questionably. "Many of them died from typhus," Dr. Larson told me recently. "Dachau's crematoriums couldn't keep up with the burning of the bodies. They did not have enough oil to keep the incinerators going. I found that a number of the victims had also died from tuberculosis. All of them were malnourished. The medical facilities were most inadequate. There was no sanitation. Two of my assistants developed TB while working with me, but apparently I'd been exposed to it so often it didn't touch me. The only infection I suffered was a cutaneous tuberculous-ulcer on one knuckle."

There were no professional autopsy rooms available, so Col. Larson and his two assistants took the best precautions they could. There wasn't even any soap available, no green soap, no Lysol; most of the time their improvised morgues were not even heated. There was no way to sterilize their surgical instruments to stop the spread of infection. One of the boys who worked with Col. Larson developed TB of the testicle and later had it amputed. His other assistant was the son of a New York City undertaker. He developed pulmonary tuberculosis and was subjected to years of treatment after the war.

Dr. Larson picks up the story:

"Dachau was a city of the dead when we got there. We found heaps of bodies outside the crematoriums, 400 to 500 bodies to a heap. Such human waste. They were horribly emaciated, horribly scarred with infected ulcers. They died in all sorts of positions: some of the legs were flexed, some not flexed, there was little muscle tissue left in the legs; many of them weighed less than 100 pounds. Most of the bodies were eastern Europeans, civilians from Poland and Rumania, most of them Jewish.

"Dachau was where they made most of the insignia worn by the German Army. I personally collected more than 1,000 Nazi emblems. A rumor going around Dachau after we got there was that many of the prisoners were poisoned. I did a lot of toxicological analysis to determine the facts and removed organs from a cross-section of about

30 or 40 bodies and sent them into Paris to the Army's First Medical Laboratory for analysis, since I lacked the proper facilities in the field. The reports came back negative. I could not find where any of these people had been poisoned. The majority died of natural diseases of one kind or another. However, we did probe into such questions as, 'What happened to those prisoners who became psychotic and developed a serious mental disease after internment at Dachau? What did the Gestapo do with them?' Well, they took those people to the crematorium. First, however, they were taken into a big windowless building next to the crematorium where the ceiling was covered with false showerheads. The victims were then ordered to strip and take a 'shower.' Outside the building, guards dropped in cyanide pellets, killing everybody inside the so-called 'shower' room. Then they'd blow the cyanide gas out and remove the bodies next door to the crematorium ovens. I think this is what happened to most of the truly psychotic prisoners and those they considered unruly and unmanageable and who, in the Gestapo's opinion, were incorrigibles. But, in my opinion, only a relatively few of the inmates I personally examined at Dachau were murdered in this manner. Still, medical facilities were totally inadequate. When people fell hopelessly ill and death was imminent, and they grew so weak they could no longer work or function, they were taken to the cyanide room for disposal. The Nazi called them 'mercy killings' because there was no hope of them getting well. Actually, the Germans considered them a liability, and extermination was the answer."

It had been almost impossible for prisoners to escape from Dachau. In addition to high barb-wire fences and trigger-happy guards, the Germans patrolled the camp area with specially-trained police dogs, mastiffs and German shepherds. They were stationed around the entire periphery of the camp. A few of them had been particularly trained to inflict punishment upon those who committed serious crimes within the camp. To make examples of them, and to deter other prisoners:

"The offender was stripped and tied to crossed boards, legs and arms spread and the animals let loose to tear the genitalia off," Dr. Larson said. "When I got there, the cages were still in place but all the dogs had been killed by the American troops who liberated Dachau. When the Americans arrived, what they saw seemed to drive them temporarily berserk. They killed the dogs and every German they could find, no matter what his story was. For a time everything was out of hand and the place was a vengeful madhouse.

"The evidence of Teutonic brutality was appalling. Outside the crematorium discarded clothing covered an area of 2,500 square feet at least 8 to 10 feet high. How many people would you have to undress to make a pile of skimpy clothing that large? This mountain of lice-infested rags was all that was left of thousands of prisoners. None of our G.I.'s would go near the pile because of typhus. You couldn't get anybody to shovel it into the furnaces to burn it up.

"Those prisoners still alive were mere scarecrows. They had gonefor days with nothing to eat, and yet, right up to the very end, the German guards were still trying to march them back and forth to work. This despite the fact that they were dropping dead from typhus with 105-degree temperatures. There were few medicines to treat the sick. They had a hospital, but the Germans couldn't take care of 10 percent of those needing medical attention."

Living conditions were deplorable. Colonel Larson's investigation revealed that approximately 100 inmates were crowded into each small barracks, 60 feet long by 17 feet wide, with virtually no ventilation.

From Col. Larson's notebook, circa 1945:

> The prisoners were forced to sleep on wooden ledges covered with straw and lay side by side with no separating

partitions. These ledges were double-decked with a space of only two feet between the upper and lower decks. There were two parallel rows of these double-deck ledges, one on each side of the room, with an aisle three feet wide down the center. Many of these barracks had no flooring. Latrine and hygienic facilities were notably inadequate. Only one small hand towel was issued to each prisoner approximately once every three months. Blankets were inadequate in number, averaging only one per person even for the winter months. Clothes were of a very poor grade of cotton-wool mixture and no overcoats were issued. Many of the prisoners had no shoes when they were liberated by the Americans. Briefly, the average diet, at the end of the war, was this:

Breakfast: A cup of weak tea or *ersatz* coffee with a small slice (75 g.) of black bread. Often nothing but the cup of tea was served. *Dinner:* The usual food was 300 to 350 cc. of a thin watery soup, prepared from potatoes and turnips with only occasionally a small amount of meat extract added for flavoring. The potatoes and turnips used in preparing these soups were of the poorest quality, often spoiled. The skins and all were utilized. *Supper:* The usual meal consisted of another 300 cc. of thin potato soup and the daily ration of 250 g. of German black bread. This bread was of the poorest quality, often very dry and mouldy. Once or twice a week a small ration of poor quality sausage or cooked horsemeat was added to the evening meal. No supplemental minerals or vitamins were provided. Daily many prisoners ate grass and other edible greens to supplement their diets. Total average daily caloric intake was 1,000 calories—far short of requirements. Since the average prisoner performed 12 hours of manual labor daily, his body required 3,000 to 4,000 calories. Thus, the extreme degree of emaciation. A very few were not so markedly emaciated. This can be explained by the fact that they worked in kitchens; a few others, for one reason or another, received special favors from the German guards. Then, too, there were still others who were able to deal on the black market for food, using as a medium of exchange the gold they had removed from the teeth of the dead.

And so there it was, an eye-witness account from inside man's Hellgates; hollow losers who'd slept with a hex.

There was one man at Dachau, a German on the staff, that Col. Larson felt should *not* have been executed. His name was Dr. Kurt Schilling. He was an internationally famous parasitologist (one who makes a scientific study of parasites). Colonel Larson had several long talks with him before he was sentenced to death by hanging.

"Dr. Schilling retired from the practice of medicine in 1932," Dr. Larson said. "During his entire professional career, commencing in 1896, he'd been a specialist in parasitology. He was for many years a professor at the University of Berlin Medical School. For 20 years he had been particularly interested in malaria and made frequent trips to Africa, Italy and the Balkans doing research on this subject. In 1936 he was summoned by Dr. Conti, German Minister of Health for the Third Reich, to appear personally before Himmler. He did this. In my conversations with Dr. Schilling at Dachau, he told me that he was ordered by Himmler to proceed to the Dachau Concentration Camp for the purpose of research in an attempt to find a method of specifically immunizing individuals against malaria because Germany was going to conquer all of Africa and it was essential to prevent malaria.

"Dr. Schilling commenced his research project at Dachau in 1936. After that he carried out experimental inoculation of healthy individuals with malaria in an attempt to develop a specific form of immunization against the disease. He admitted to me that between the years 1936 and 1945 he inoculated some 2,000 prisoners with malaria. He did not personally pick the subjects, he said, except that he'd request 30 to 40 individuals at a time and specify they be healthy. The medical supervisor at Dachau would select those people to be inoculated, send the list to Berlin to have it approved by higher authority and, when the list was returned, those who were chosen were then turned over to

Dr. Schilling at the Dachau Hospital where he'd reserved two floors specifically for them.

"Two methods of malarial inoculation were used. The first was by means of human blood infected by malaria, and the second was by means of using infected mosquitoes and permitting them to bite the patients. He told me that he'd used only benign Tertian malaria but that he had used some 40 different strains of this parasite. The first group of experiments consisted of inoculating his patients with malaria, permitting them to have some varying numbers of chills ranging in number from 2 to 14, and then curing them, or attempting to cure them with the available drugs, Atabrine and Quinine. This was done in an attempt to determine whether or not the facilities of cure differed, depending upon the number of attacks of fever. The second set of experiments consisted of inoculating healthy people with the malaria and when the prodromal symptoms developed, to start treatment before chills and fever had occurred. Some of these people were inoculated several times, and when the initial prodromal symptoms appeared, they were treated. Dr. Schilling further told me that after several inoculations treated before the chills and fever developed, that subsequently he was unable to infect these people with malaria of the same strain. He believed that he had produced a latent form of the disease in these patients which gave them immunity against an acute attack of malaria, by this particular strain of the parasite. He showed me his records to substantiate his second group of experiments.

"The third group of experiments were conducted using a drug known as 'Pyramidon.' This suppressed the fever in malaria but did not cure the disease. Here Dr. Schilling was attempting to develop a therapy which would lead to immunity and at the same time not subject the individual to the rigors of chills and fever. Pyramidon had the bad feature of depressing the white blood cell count and, in my opinion, ran the risk of causing some deaths due to a medical condition known as *Agranulocytosis*. Dr. Schilling frankly confessed that he did not believe this third experiment was the answer to the treatment of malaria, because of the danger accompanied by the use of this drug Pyramidon.

"On March 14 an order came down from Berlin to destroy all records of these medical experiments. At the time the order was issued, Dr. Schilling was in the hospital himself, recovering from an operation upon his prostate. He told me that while many of his records were destroyed by his assistants who carried out the order from Berlin, he still had many papers intact at his home.

"It was very difficult to know where to draw the line as to whether or not Dr. Schilling was a war criminal. Certainly he fell in that category inasmuch as he had subjected people involuntarily to experimental malaria inoculations, which, even though they did not produce many deaths, could very well have produced serious illness in many of the patients. He defended himself by saying he did all this work by order from higher authority; in fact, Himmler himself.

"In my report, I wrote: 'In view of all he has told me, this man, in my opinion, should be considered a war criminal, but that he should be permitted to write up the results of his experiments and turn them over to Allied medical personnel for what they are worth. Dr. Schilling is an eminent scientist of world-wide renown who has conducted a most important group of experiments; their value cannot be properly ascertained until he has put them into writing for medical authorities to study. The criminal acts have already been committed, and since they have been committed, if it were possible to derive some new knowledge concerning immunity to malaria from these acts, it would be yet another crime not to permit this man to finish documenting the results of his years of research.'

"But my attempt to save Dr. Schilling's life failed. Our High Command felt it had to make a public example of him—most of the other high-ranking Nazis connected with Dachau had already been executed—and made his wife watch the hanging. I did everything I could to stop it. I implored our military government not to pass sentence on him until he'd had a fair hearing, because I was just beginning to win his confidence, to get through to him. Looking back, I am sure that the execution of Dr. Schilling deprived the world of some very valuable scientific information—no matter how distasteful his research and experimentation may have been."

There were other medical experiments conducted at Dachau—stupid, ghoulish experiments which personified the insane, systematic brutality of Hitler's Third Reich. As the shocked, uprooted prisoners arrived by rail, the first person they saw was usually an officer impeccably turned out in a dress SS uniform. Placing himself between the rows of new arrivals, he decided their fate: a flick of a thin metal rod, held by a white-gloved hand, to the left meant immediate death in the gas ovens; to the right meant life—but what a life. Most of the prisoners would survive for only a few more weeks, doing hard labor on starvation rations or serving as guinea pigs in a series of experiments. One test was to determine how long a person could survive in cold water. This experiment was requested by the German air force, because their planes were flying across the North Sea on their bombing runs to England. That water is like Puget Sound in the State of Washington—banker's-heart cold.

"A Dr. Raschau was in charge of this work and had escaped from Dachau before we got there, but we found the record of his experiments," Dr. Larson recalls. "They were most inept compared to Dr. Schilling's, much less scientific. What they would do would be to tie up a prisoner and immerse him in cold water until his body temperature reduced to 28 degrees centigrade (82.4 degrees Fahrenheit), when the poor soul would, of course, die. These experiments were started in August, 1942, but Raschau's technique improved. By February, 1943 he was able to report that 30 persons were chilled to 27 and 29 degrees centigrade, their hands and feet frozen white, and their bodies 'rewarmed' by a hot bath. According to some reports, the victims had been rewarmed by animal heat. That is, he was surrounded with the naked bodies of warm women until his frozen body responded to his environment sufficiently to have sexual intercourse.

"They also dressed the subjects in different types of insulated clothing before putting them in freezing water, to see how long it took them to die. They murdered a lot of people that way. I never saw Dr. Raschau or got a chance to interview him. He was a man in his 40s or 50s and a typical hard-nose Nazi. He was something like Dr. Josef Mengele, the SS physician, known as the Angel of Death, who sent millions to the gas chambers at Auschwitz-Birkenau and killed thousands more in mad genetic exmeriments. Dr. Mengele, for example, tried to turn the eyes of children blue by painfully injecting them with dye.

"On the other hand, Dr. Schilling, who was 72, should have lived. He never tried to run. He stayed at Dachau and made a full statement of his work to me; he cooperated in every way, and was the only one who told the truth and gave us all of the information on Dr. Raschau."

After 10 days at Dachau, working almost the clock around each day, Col. Larson reached a state of exhaustion he had never before known. He passed the point of known weakness and from then on he lived in a sort of waking sleep. He kept on, however, because the work had to be done. There were times when he could not remember accurately when he had eaten last or when he had last slept. The snatched food sitting heavily on the stomach, the stench, the flies, the mutilated bodies. Eventually it all worked itself into indefinable tapestry of yesterday is tomorrow and today is yesterday. Dachau is Kauffring and Buchenwald is Landsburg and when will they ever reach the end of all these starved bodies and, God, he was so tired.

The result was that Col. Larson finally grew befogged. He was mentally as well as physically drained. All feeling had left him. He looked absently out across those fields of the dead, seeing only faintly and not really wanting to see at all. The human wreckage. The awful waste and senseless destruction of war.

At Dachau Col. Larson's work—the profile of the prisoner population that his autopsies projected—indicated that only a small percentage of the deaths were due to medical experimentation on humans. It indicated that most of the victims died from so-called "natural causes" at the time; that is, of disease brought on by malnutrition and filth which are the handmaidens of war.

A team of Army lawyers spent three days with Col. Larson taking his depositions. He made it perfectly clear he could not find it in him to indict the whole German people for the Nazi crimes. Though Dachau was only a short ride from Munich, Col. Larson sincerely believed that most of the people in the city had no idea of what was going on behind the Dachau barbed wire.

"The security around all of the camps I worked in was so tight that at each one I found German civilians living less than a mile away who had no idea of what was going on inside," Dr. Larson said. "The only ones who knew what was happening were the Nazis and those Nazi sympathizers who had business inside. The rest of the German populace was kept in ignorance, possibly to keep them from rising up against Hitler and his henchmen. While I was at Dachau, thousands of German civilians were taken through the prison and shown what had gone on; they were horrified. I personally talked to many of them, and I tell you, you cannot fake the reaction they had!"

The Body in Striped Pajamas

AMERICANS are people who read millions of who-done-its a month and never really believe them—because we, as a nation, make the worst damn spies in all of history. *Watergate?*

What we seem to read for is the appearance of a mastermind who quite unexpectedly stands up and calmly says, "The button is from Arbutnot's vest—therefore, the butler did it."

Sophisticated. Smart stuff.

Well, there are no masterminds in the crime detection business, merely the fact, as in any business, that some minds are sharper than others. As in international espionage, crime detection is a matter usually of putting together the small, puzzling bits and pieces contributed by many sleuths. In Los Angeles, Chicago and New York it's a fact that there have been at various times hundreds of professional detectives detailed to running down one laundry mark.

Dr. Larson is one of a small group of highly qualified physician-surgeons who can, given a dead body as yet undisturbed by other investigators, tell what caused the death, and he can put the authorities on the road to identification. With those two basic questions answered, it becomes a matter of interrogation of all who *could* have committed the act—until the only person left is the one who *did* it.

On Monday, October 23, 1961 the Atlanta, Georgia police department put out a call to homicide detectives J.F. Inman and L.W. Bradley to phone headquarters. When they phoned back, they were told that a Dr. Lester Rumble had contacted headquarters asking for someone to check the residence of Dr. Elmer Lee Fry, at 3645 Peachtree Road, Apartment 100. Dr. Fry had not been heard from for a day and a half, and it was unusual for him not to report in before 9:15 a.m. daily.

"I tried Dr. Fry's apartment but received no answer," Dr. Rumble told the police. So Officers Inman and Bradley went to the apartment and got the residence manager to open up Dr. Fry's front door with a pass key. They found Dr. Fry lying face-down on the floor in the doorway between the living room and the bedroom. His head was buried in a thick, shaggy-pile rug. He had been dead for some time. There was no sign of violence, no wounds other than a bruise on the right cheek. But there was blood and mucus running from the mouth and nose. Dr. Rumble arrived and said that the last person to hear from Dr. Fry was his ex-wife who had talked to him on the phone the previous Saturday night. Other than that, nothing.

At the Fulton County Morgue an autopsy was performed on the body because when death occurs *not* under the care of a physician the law requires autopsy:

EXTERNAL EXAMINATION.

"Clothing—The body was clad in striped cotton pajamas which were without remarkable features (tears, stains or other defects). These garments were removed and the body was washed and all areas of the skin were examined with a hand lens.

Body—The body was that of an adult white male, normally developed and adequately nourished. The external appearance of the body was consistent with the stated age of 40. Rigor mortis was firmly established throughout with the arms in a position of partial flexion. Lividity was prominent and fixed in the skin of the anterior aspects of the body. There were irregular areas of pressure pallor in the regions of the shoulders, thighs and left cheek. There were no injuries, signs of external violence or marks on the external surface, except for an irregular pressure mark in the skin overlying the prominence of the left cheek bone. This area was dark purple and had a prominent cross-hatch pattern of the involved skin which was suggestive of the coarse weave of fabric. The hair of the head was greying and cut short. The eyes were unremarkable. The pupils were circular and of equal diameter (approximately 3 mm). The corneas were clear and the orbits were firm. The oral and nasal cavities contained small amounts of dark-brown mucinous material. A small amount of this material was present on the lower lip. The teeth were normal and the oral mucosa was intact. There was no external evidence of natural disease, no gross skeletal deformity or other abnormality.

Date 12-6-61
Signed: Tom Dillon.

Now, here's another report by Dr. Tom Dillon made *after* the initial external examination:

AUTOPSY OR INTERNAL EXAMINATION OF ELMER L. FRY—

The usual Y-shaped incision was made to open the body cavities and the subcutaneous soft tissues were unremarkable. The bony thorax was intact. The chest plate was removed by incising the costal cartilages. The internal organs maintained their normal relationship one to another. There was no excess fluid in any body cavity.

CARDIOVASCULAR SYSTEM: The heart weighed 278 grams. It was of normal external configuration and examination of the myocardium, cardiac chambers, valves and coronary arteries disclosed no gross abnormalities. The aorta and its major branches were unremarkable. The blood within the cardiovascular system was cyanotic. There were numerous small soft blood clots present within the heart.

RESPIRATORY SYSTEM: The organs of the neck were removed enbloc and were unremarkable. There was no obstruction of the upper airway. The hyoid bone, laryngeal cartilages and cervical spine were intact. The thyroid gland was unremarkable. The lungs had a combined weight of 610 grams. There was congestion and subcrepitence of the anterior segments of both lungs. The remaining segments of both lungs were well aerated and unremarkable. The larger bronchi contained small amounts of red-brown mucus, but were otherwise unremarkable.

GASTROINTESTINAL SYSTEM: Unremarkable throughout. The stomach contained an estimated 100 ml. of turbid olive-green fluid. The intestinal contents were normal.

LIVER AND BILLARY SYSTEM: The liver weighed 1300 grams. The external surface and multiple cut sections were unremarkable except for moderate congestion. The gall bladder and extra hepatic bile ducts were negative.

PANCREAS, SPLEEN, AND ADRENALS: Unremarkable.

GENITOURINARY SYSTEM: The kidneys were estimated to weigh 125 grams each. The external surfaces were smooth and the cut sections of both kidneys were unremarkable. The ureters and urinary bladder were negative. There was approximately 75 ml. of clear amber urine in the bladder. The external genitalia, testes and prostate were unremarkable.

HEAD: The scalp was incised and reflected in the usual manner and was negative. There was no hemorrhage into the galea. The cranial vault was intact and was opened with the customary saw-cuts. There was no intracranial hemorrhage. The cerebral blood vessels were unre-

markable. The brain weighed 1610 grams. It was of normal external configuration.
Date 12-6-61
Signed: Tom Dillon, M.D.
Medical Examiner

The upshot was that Medical Examiner Dillon was unable to determine the cause of death and signed his report to that effect. But there was about $1,000,000 worth of insurance involved if Doctor Fry's death was found to be accidental. When the widow brought suit, the insurance companies opened battery fire calling in Dr. Milton Halpern, the celebrated New York City Medical Examiner (and an old friend of Dr. Larson's); Dr. Francis Camps, the Internationally-known Scotland Yard pathologist (another friend of Dr. Larson's); and Dr. John T. Godwin, Professor of Pathology at Emory University. The three were called in by the insurance companies to serve as expert witnesses. They had all gone over the Atlanta Medical Examiner's autopsy report, and none of them had come up with a positive cause of death. They had made sections (prepared tissue to be examined under the microscope) of the liver and the heart and given depositions that *implied* that death had been caused by a ventricular fibrillation affecting the nervous conduction system of the heart (medical vernacular for a frequent cause of death in chronic alcoholics). To substantiate this a slide showing a little fatty infiltration of the liver, to prove that Dr. Fry was an alcoholic, was placed in exhibit.

Backed by the depositions of the distinguished pathologists, the insurance companies' position, in summarization, read like this:

1. Dr. Fry's liver was abnormally fatty.
2. Alcoholics have fatty livers.
3. Therefore, Dr. Fry was an alcoholic.
4. Dr. Fry died.
5. Therefore, he died the death of an alcoholic.

Enter Dr. Larson...

In the spring of '62, he received a long-distance call at Tacoma General Hospital. His secretary, Esther Short, said, "Dr. Larson, an attorney from Atlanta, Georgia is on the line."

Dr. Larson picked up the phone. "Yes?"

A very thick-tongued Southern drawl said: "Dr. Lahson, this is Mistah Hah-mon."

"Who?"

"Mistah Hah-mon. Harmon. Nolan B. Hah-mon. May I come out and see yo-all?"

"What about?"

"If ah tell yoh, yoh won't talk to me."

He really had Dr. Larson's attention now.

"When do you want to come?"

"Ah'll fly out tonight and see yoh in the morning."

At precisely 11 a.m. the following day, Nolan B. Harmon, attorney at law, a very fine-looking Southern gentleman, impeccably dressed, walked into Dr. Larson's office and took a seat in the far corner.

"Why wouldn't you tell me on the phone what you want?" Dr. Larson began.

"It's a very long story," Mr. Harmon said. "It involves some professional friends of yours—people I am sure you wouldn't want to lock horns with in a court of law."

"That doesn't make any difference," Dr. Larson told him. "I always form my own opinion—and testify on the basis of what I believe to be the truth."

"Well, I have depositions here I want you to read."

He opened his briefcase and pulled out four depositions. The first one was from Dr. Milton Helpern; the second, a letter from Dr. Francis Camps, of London, England; the third, a deposition from Dr. Thomas Dillon, Atlanta Medical Examiner; and the last, a deposition from Dr. John T. Godwin.

Dr. Larson spent the following hour reading this

material. When he finished, he turned to Harmon and said, "Now!!!"

"Before you say you will not accept the case," broke in Harmon, "*please*, let me give you my side of it."

Dr. Larson relaxed, sank back in his chair.

Mr. Harmon continued. "I have been informed that you are a very competent forensic pathologist and I am here because I believe you can come up with the correct solution to the case after you've heard and seen all the facts."

Whereupon Mr. Harmon elaborated in great detail all of the known facts—as well as his personal investigation—of the strange circumstances surrounding the death of Dr. Fry.

"I do not believe Dr. Fry was an alcoholic," Harmon said. "I do not believe alcohol was a cause of his death. I do not believe the marks on the body were postmortem or pressure phenomena. I don't believe, up to now, *anyone* knows the true cause of death. But whatever it was, there must be a scientific explanation—and that this explanation will probably prove *accidental* death."

Very briefly, that was what Mr. Harmon told Dr. Larson, who told him to leave the material with him for more study. They made a dinner date for that evening.

Dr. Larson gave the case a lot of thought and study. He finally came up with a reasonable solution to the case, based on the medical evidence, the photographs, and the police and Mr. Harmon's investigation. All this evidence seemed to clearly indicate that the cause of death was postural asphyxiation. He then studied all available literature on the subject; in addition, he telephoned his son, Charles Philip Larson, Jr. M.D., at the University of California Medical School where he was an Associate Professor of Anesthesiology. After the facts were presented to him, Dr. Larson, Jr. agreed with his father that Dr. Fry probably died an asphyxial death. He buttressed this opinion by describing a colored motion picture he recently made in the operating room of a patient undergoing haemorroidectomy (the surgical removal of piles). This operation requires the subject to be face down.

"As the film progresses," Dr. Larson, Jr. told his dad, "you can see the patient becoming increasingly more cynotic (getting bluer and bluer) as his posture curtailed his air intake. He was slowly smothering by virtue of the position of his body. Had it not been changed, he'd have died."

Dr. Larson, Sr. went to dinner that evening thoroughly convinced that his theory was, in fact, *the fact.*

He told Mr. Harmon, "I've decided to take the case. I think I know why Dr. Fry died."

Mr. Harmon was very excited.

"I knew you'd come up with the right answer," he said. "That's why I followed my hunch and flew all the way out here from Atlanta. Mrs. Fry and her children are going to be very happy. They really need the money. Dr. Fry did not leave them very well off. Dr. Larson, would you be willing to go to Atlanta to make your own investigation and testify?"

"Under the circumstances, I feel it's my obligation," Dr. Larson said.

When Dr. Larson was called in on the case, approximately a year after the fact of Dr. Fry's death, he went to Atlanta and examined the scene, as well as he could at that late date, through photographs of the body and of the surroundings and from reports from the initial investigating officers, J.F. Inman and L.W. Bradley.

Dr. Larson's pencilled notes, made at the time, revealed the following:

> "Bachelor apt., but clean, neat. *Alcoholics are sloppy.* No drugs or liquor in apt. Bed clean. Peculiar position of arms (right forearm under chest, left forearm under abdomen, indicating they'd doubled under as the body pitched down). Bruise on left cheek. Bruise on left side of nose. Tooth mark on left lower lip. Found lying on the floor, face-

down, between bedroom and bathroom, his knees off the rug, his face on it."

When Dr. Larson looked at those old notes recently, his mind flashed back 15 years—with total recall.

"All the doors of this apartment were locked from the inside, the windows were all locked and there was positively no evidence that anybody had broken in," Dr. Larson told me. "The problem was to determine why this man died. Three eminent forensic pathologists had been unable to come up with a positive cause of death, so I *had* to. I couldn't just go into court with the negative assertion that he was *not* a chronic alcoholic; therefore, alcoholism could *not* be the cause of his death. You have to be precise with a jury—*factual.*"

Dr. Larson read the depositions of the defense pathologists. They had gone over all the work that Medical Examiner Dr. Dillon had done in Atlanta. They had made sections of the liver and the heart, and on the basis of the sections, Dr. Milton Halpern gave a deposition that, in effect, said that Dr. Fry died of ventricular fibrillation of the heart, due to chronic alcoholism affecting the nervous conduction system of the heart; this even though there was no alcohol in Dr. Fry's blood at the time he died. To prove his point, Dr. Halpern showed a little fatty infiltration of the liver.

Dr. Larson had a lot of evidence that Nolan B. Harmon had gathered which indicated the deceased had not been a chronic alcoholic; certainly his apartment was not that of a chronic alcoholic. Obviously the Atlanta police had given up on the idea of a homicide. Nobody could have gotten in and relocked all the windows and doors from the inside, with the bolt shot on the front door, and got outside again.

"There was a hemorrhagic area (blood congested beneath the skin) on the side of the face of Dr. Fry that bothered me slightly from the beginning—a large bruise on his left forehead and lesions (bruises) on his knees," Dr.

Larson recollected. "But these, I was certain, were impact bruises.

"Against the healthy coffers of Equitable Life, Metropolitan Life and Lumberman's Mutual Casualty Company—all three of which were fighting double-indemnity liability on contention that Dr. Fry did *not* die accidently—there was a cool million dollars to guarantee the future of Dr. Fry's two small, and otherwise penniless children. And there was my slowly growing conviction that Dr. Fry *did* die accidentally."

Go back, now, with Dr. Larson.

In the sworn statement of the Medical Examiner of Fulton County who had performed the autopsy, one item was of particular significance. There had been 75 milliliters of clear amber urine in the bladder. This indicated to Dr. Larson that Elmer Fry had gotten up from bed to go to the bathroom.

"Now a man who knows his home premises well, does not need a light to find his way around at night," Dr. Larson pointed out. "Further, if he has sensitive eyes he will not put a light on. Dr. Fry had sensitive eyes, hence his apartment was tightly curtained to admit *no* light at all. The body was found on a line between the bedroom and the bathroom. I worked it out in my mind that Dr. Fry had gotten up and, on his way to the bathroom, had, in the darkness, tripped on the loose rug and, in falling, had hit his head upon the corner of the table. This knocked him unconscious. With his face and mouth pushed down into the wadded-up rug, he had died of postural asphyxia (smothering to death by virtue of the position of his body). Postural asphyxia is known to a few pathologists, but very little has been written on the subject—and there are only a very few authenticated cases. But most anesthesiologists (doctors of medicine who specialize in surgical sedation) know about it, because whenever surgery requires a patient to be upon the table face down, the anesthesiologist has to be alert every moment to protect the patient's airways or he'll die on the table of postural asphyxia."

Ask a fan what the great American sport is, and he will probably give one of three answers: football, baseball or basketball. In each case he would be wrong. The true national sport is the *Law*, and the contest Americans love best is the one in the courtroom, where lives are at stake and vast sums can be won or lost on a lawyer's forward motion.

The Dr. Fry case went to trial finally and lasted for two weeks. Dr. Larson was permitted to sit in on all of it, for the plaintiff was allowed one doctor to sit in, as were the insurance companies. They chose Dr. King, the chief medical director for Metropolitan Life.

Following the reading of Dr. Francis Camps' deposition, Dr. Halpern was called to the stand. He was one of the best expert medical witnesses in the world. Going to court as an expert witness takes a bit of doing. Whereas Dr. Larson always has had a deep respect for the jury system in America, he does confess that the ponderosity of a lot of the procedure amuses him. But as long as he gets enjoyment from it, he usually tries to give some in return. Within the spectrum of facts, he puts on the best show he can come up with to stimulate his ingenuity.

"You are aware, no doubt, of how opposing lawyers snarl and growl and browbeat each other all morning in court and then, arm in arm, go out to lunch together?" Dr. Larson said. "Well, Milton Halpern was a close friend of mine, and I knew his worth thoroughly and his deadliness on the witness stand. So I pulled his cork. When he was walking down the aisle to take the stand, Nolan Harmon, the 'li'l ole Georgia lawyer,' as he first described himself to me, turned to me and said, 'What shall I ask him in cross examination? What shall I do? He's a big caliber New York medical gun. He can snow me under.' On a quick hunch I told Mr. Harmon not to take on an elephant. 'Ask him instead,' I told him, 'if he's the New York Medical Examiner. Ask him where he went to school, how his wife is, who's the governor of his state. Ask him where he lives, how long has he been practicing medicine—and then thank him and let him step down.' I don't know how much of the one year of law I took at Gonzaga University has stayed with me, and I don't actually believe that study of the law is necessary to the practice of forensic pathology, but I did not want Dr. Halpern to go back into the substance of his deposition and clutter up the record with a discussion of chronic alcoholism, ventricular fibrillation and the nervous conduction system of the heart, for a jury can stand just so much of the technical jargon of expert testimony in any field—and no more. Besides, Dr. Halpern was a formidable and most convincing man on the stand, and I wanted him out of the way."

Which is what Mr. Harmon did. The coast was clear now for Dr. Larson to be called to the stand as the plaintiff's rebuttal witness. His testimony covered two full days. It went like this:

DIRECT EXAMINATION:

Mr. Harmon: Doctor, would you state your name for the record, please?

A: My name is Charles P. Larson. L-a-r-s-o-n.

Q: Where are you from?

A: Tacoma, Washington.

Q: Let me ask you this, Doctor. You have been sitting at counsel table with us during the trial. How did you happen to be sitting there?

A: Well, I was sitting there principally because you asked me to sit there. I arrived here to testify and you asked me if I would mind sitting at the table, and I did so at your request.

Q: Other than being a witness in this case do you have any financial interest in the outcome of the case or anything like that?

A: None whatsoever.

Q: All right, sir. Let me ask you this. I want to ask you some questions about your qualifications, Doctor. First of all, where did you take your undergraduate education?

A: I graduated from Gonzaga University in Spokane with a Bachelor of Arts Degree and a major in chemistry in 1931.

Q: Where did you take your medical training?

A: I took my medical training at McGill University in Montreal, Quebec, and I graduated in 1936 with a degree of Doctor of Medicine and a Master of Surgery.

Q: Now, where did you take your internship?

A: I took my internship at the Pierce County Hospital in Tacoma, Washington.

Q: Did you specialize in any particular branch of medicine, Doctor?

A: Yes. I specialized in pathology and in forensic pathology.

Q: And are you certified by any boards in pathology of the American Medical Association?

A: Yes. I am certified by the American Board of Pathology, in the field of Pathologic Anatomy and in the field of Forensic Pathology.

Q: Now, what are you doing currently, Doctor?

A: Currently I am the senior partner of a group of eight pathologists who practice in my community, and we serve a number of hospitals. We have some private laboratories. My particular specialty, and I spend the bulk of my time in this, is in the field of forensic pathology, although I still do a generous amount of general pathology and clinical pathology, but the bulk of my time is spent in the field of forensic pathology.

Q: What is forensic pathology?

A: Forensic pathology deals with the application of the same principles you really study in pathologic anatomy, except they deal with the application of these principles to the law and to the solution of problems of death in which there is some question about how this individual died or what the sequence of events was and how a person died. The work of a medical examiner, for example, like Dr. Halpern testified here, is the work of a forensic pathologist. That is what a forensic pathologist is. He is a man who conducts investigations as to why people die under unknown, suspicious or circumstances which are not known clearly to the physician prior to the time of death.

Q: Now, what is the College of American Pathologists, Doctor?

A: The College of American Pathologists is the largest

single organization of pathologists in the world, and it is a scientific body of pathologists who group themselves together for scientific reasons and other reasons.

Q: Are you a member of that?

A: Yes, sir. I am a member, and I served as president for two years.

Q: Well, Doctor, let me ask you this. Were you in service during World War II?

A: Yes, sir.

Q: Were you in any particular theater?

A: Yes, I was in the European Theater of operations.

Q: Did you do any pathology work at the close of World War II?

A: Well, I might say, Mr. Harmon, that all I did during World War II was pathology, but the last several months of the time I spent in the European Theater was—I was engaged in investigating war crimes, and I was the chief pathologist for the War Crimes Team for southern Germany.

Q: Have you ever served in any consulting position?

A: Many of them, yes.

Q: Have you ever served the Armed Forces Institute of Pathology in any sort of consulting capacity?

A: Yes, as a consultant in forensic pathology.

Q: Have you ever done any work with any police departments or police department crime laboratories in a consulting capacity?

A: Yes. This is the only salaried position which I hold at the present time, and I have held this for many years, and that is that I am the Consultant and Pathologic Director of the Tacoma Police Crime Laboratory, and I still hold this position, and I hold the rank of captain in our police department.

Q: Have you written any papers?

A: Yes, sir.

Q: Could you give us an idea of about how many?

A: Well, I couldn't tell you exactly, but I made a bibliography of them a few minutes ago and at that time there were over sixty papers I had published in the American literature.

Q: Have you written any books?

A: I wrote a teaching manual on the subject of neuropathology which I mentioned earlier.

Q: Now, Doctor, you mentioned a few minutes ago that a great deal of your time is spent in investigating unusual deaths. Where, in terms of geographical area, do you go in investigating these deaths?

A: Well, I have gone pretty much all over the country, but if you mean personally investigating the death itself, I have personally investigated unusual deaths in most of the western states, and this would include the states of Nevada, Idaho, Montana, Oregon, Washington and Alaska.

Q: Now, Doctor, how do you go about investigating? Just give us an idea of the general procedure, how do you go about investigating an unusual death?

A: Well, I am kind of a nut on this, Mr. Harmon, and I have written papers on this, so I feel free to talk about it. I feel that it is a responsibility of a forensic pathologist or a person who practices this specialty to go to the scene of where the body is found, and that you must go there and you must observe this body before it is disturbed or before anything is done with the body. This is very important for many reasons. It gives you a chance to see the exact circumstances in which the body was found. It gives the pathologist who has peculiar knowledge about certain things an opportunity to pick up evidence that might be missed by police departments, and this is very often extremely important in criminal cases, pick up trace evidence, minute pieces of evidence that would be missed by police departments and even by crime laboratories and organizations such as this.

So, Mr. Harmon, I have made it my practice now for a number of years, and I repeat, I have written papers on this and I feel very strongly about it, under the circumstances I will not accept a case to investigate it unless I am called to the scene before the body is disturbed and before the body is moved. I have been called away as far as Alaska in which they have sealed the house and sealed the place where the body was found, left it undisturbed until I was able to get an airplane to go to, say, Juneau, Alaska, and investigate this case.

I have a very strong feeling that if you are going to do a

proper forensic pathologic examination of a body in which there are found strange or unusual circumstances, that it is most necessary for the pathologist to be at the scene and to see and know of his own first-hand knowledge the situation and also be able to determine and pick up what evidence he would see at the scene in order to solve this particular problem. Actually, in recent years I have refused to take cases where the body has been moved.

Q: All right, sir. Now, I want to ask you some questions about some of the exhibits that are in the evidence. First of all, in connection with this particular case have you had an opportunity, first, to examine Plaintiffs' Exhibit 8?

THE COURT:

What is Plaintiffs' Exhibit 8, the autopsy report?

MR. HARMON:

It is the autopsy report, Your Honor.

THE WITNESS:

Yes, I have examined this autopsy report in great detail.

MR. HARMON:

Q: Well, I am going to ask you some specific questions about it in a few minutes, but have you also had an opportunity to examine Plaintiffs' Exhibit 9 and Plaintiffs' Exhibit 11, this one here, and 10 and 13?

A: Yes. I have not only examined these pictures, I have even placed these pictures under varying degrees of microscopic magnification to study them.

Q: Have you examined the slides which are in evidence as Plaintiffs' Exhibit 14?

A: Yes, sir.

Q: And have you examined these photographs, Defendants' Exhibits 1 and 2?

A: Yes.

Q: Now, would you come down before the jury, please, sir, just a minute and let me ask you a question about some of these photographs?

A: Yes. (Whereupon, the witness left the witness stand and went down before the jury.)

MR. HARMON:

Q: Now, this is, first of all, Plaintiffs' Exhibit No. 11. Now, let me show you that and particularly the mark on the left cheek of the body there, and let me ask you whether or not you have any opinion as to what that mark is.

A: I most certainly do have an opinion as to what that mark is, yes.

Q: And what is that opinion?

A: In my opinion this mark is a bruise.

Q: Now, Doctor, tell us—

A: May I explain why?

Q: Yes, sir, please do.

A: My reasons for this are several. You have heard, as I have heard, in this courtroom the argument as to whether this is a bruise or a pressure mark. I have many reasons why I believe this is not a pressure mark. First of all, a pressure mark would not look to me as it does in this picture. Before I get to the other reasons why I say this is not a pressure mark, I do want to preface my remarks to the jury and be ultimately fair about this and say that the only way that anybody can look at a picture like this and determine whether or not this is a bruise or a pressure mark, it would be pure opinion, really. There is nobody in the world who can look at a picture like this and say, sure, it is unequivocally a bruise or it is unequivocally a pressure mark. The ultimate proof of what this is would have been to have taken a little piece of tissue here, it could have been a very thin one, a little tiny thin sliver of tissue out of there and made a microscopic slide of it, and we wouldn't have had all this argument as to whether this was a bruise or whether this was a pressure mark. There would have been no question. Had we a microcsopic section to look at under the microscope and see whether or not there was hemorrhage, whether or not there were changes in the cellular tissue underneath this, which would have distinguished very quickly and very readily between a pressure mark and a bruise.

Now, I have many reasons for saying this is not a pressure mark, because I have observed many pressure marks in people over the years, and I would say this to you, that if this is a pressure mark, why do we not have a pressure mark in other places on this body?

Q: You are referring now, Doctor to—

A: I am referring to this pressure—this mark here on the cheek.

Q: But you were just talking about—

A: I am talking about another picture here. You handed me three pictures. Here I have a full-length picture of the body, and we have the right arm underneath the body. Now if you will feel your elbow, you have very little tissues supporting your elbow. In other words, the bone is right under the elbow bone, and if a man has all of his weight lying on the weight of that elbow for a long period of time when he was alive and he didn't move, why didn't he have a pressure mark here? If he lay in this position with his knees, and you can feel your knees have very little protection, certainly no more than the side of your face, and if he is lying here with his knees on a hard floor, not even a rug, why doesn't he have a pressure mark there?

I mean, I have observed many, many pressure marks, but I have seen in these cases that there is not a single pressure mark. In order to get a pressure mark, you have to presume many other things. In other words, you have to have many other things that have happened to this particular individual.

Now, a person who lies on the floor like this who had good circulation, in other words, his heart is beating normally and the blood is normally flowing through his body, he doesn't get pressure marks just from lying on a floor.

I am sure you can go to sleep on a floor like this and lie there all night, if your heart is beating correctly, and you are not going to get any pressure marks from that. We get pressure marks when there is very poor circulation, the heart isn't beating well over a long period of time. This is what produces pressure marks. In my opinion this man died rather suddenly. He didn't lie here for a long period of time. And, secondly, I don't think he had poor heart action for a long period of time. You have to have these things in order to get a pressure mark. For that reason I contend that although certainly from this picture nobody can say what this is, I contend from the other reasoning I have given you this is not a pressure mark and that this does, in fact, represent a bruise.

Q: All right, sir. Now, let me ask you this. In a situation like this do you have an opinion, looking at that body there, as to whether or not the bruise you have testified about was caused prior to death or caused after death?

A: Yes, sir, I have an opinion about that, too.

Q: What is that opinion?

A: I have the opinion that this is definitely caused before death. I don't know of any post mortem bruising phenomenon that would look like this in a picture that would occur, say, after death. In other words, if somebody walked in and picked up his head and hit his head on the floor after he was dead, he would cause post mortem bruises—but I don't think they would assume this color. Sometimes they are a little difficult to distinguish, but in my opinion this occurred before death.

Q: Doctor, if somebody hit me in the face on the cheekbone hard with their fist and then, oh, let's say, a minute later I was killed, somebody put a bullet through my heart, could a bruise form, could discoloration form in this cheek after I was dead, or would that be impossible, in your judgment?

A: You have allowed a minute here. In one minute there can be hemorrhage, there can be considerable hemorrhage if somebody hits you on the side of the cheek. Within one minute you can develop considerable hemorrhage into the tissues which, after a period of time, after a few hours after death, the blood breaks down, whether you are alive or dead, and this thing would become black and blue just as it does during life, and the same cycles occur in the blood which has already gotten out into the tissues from this blow, whether you are dead or alive after it happens. In other words, hemorrhages in the tissue will discolor after death. Did I answer your question?

Q: Yes, sir.

(Whereupon, the witness returned to the witness stand.)

MR. HARMON:

Q: Doctor, I want you to assume the information contained in the—take into consideration the information contained in the coroner's report, the information contained in the photographs that I have shown you, the information contained in the slides, and all the photographs, and I will ask you if you have any opinion, assuming all those facts, if you have any opinion as to the cause of the death of this person.

A: Yes, I do.

Q: What is that opinion?

A: It is my opinion that Dr. Fry suffered a traumatic injury to his cheek, which is visible in these photographs. It is further my opinion from the photographs and the position of the body that this man fell, the rug is rumpled up, the head is in a most unusual position, the arms in an unusual position under the body, so it is my opinion that this man fell, that either prior to falling or due to falling on the rug he sustained an injury to his left cheek. It is further my opinion that because of the position in which the body was found and because of the extent of this bruise which I think could well be sufficient to produce unconsciousness, that this man suffered from what I would call hypoxia or postural asphyxia, and that this, in my opinion, at least, is the immediate cause of death in this individual.

Q: Now—

A: I haven't given you all the reasons why I think this way.

Q: Go ahead, sir, and give us some more, if you will.

A: Well, first of all, this man if found in a position which is most unnatural, and in my opinion, after studying the autopsy, I don't think that we are able to rule out the obstruction of an airway. I wish I could sit here and tell you that forensic pathologists could always determine whether or not the airway is obstructed, but, unfortunately, I can't tell you this. I don't think it is possible in all instances for a forensic pathologist or anybody else doing an autopsy, particularly after a body has been moved, to tell you whether or not during life this airway was obstructed or not. Sure, you can move the body back to the morgue and change the position of the body and change the position of the things as they were during life, and you might be able to determine this.

In a circumstance like this where a man is found dead on a floor, if you are looking for an obstructed airway and you are going to determine for sure whether this man died of asphyxia and he had an obstructed airway, the only logical method of determining this would be to bring a piece of apparatus with you and see whether or not you get air in or out of the lungs before you turned him over and before you moved him and before you disturbed him. I don't think there is any autopsy technique in the world that can establish unequivocally beyond a doubt one way or the other whether a person has an obstructed airway of the type that we are talking of here. Now, remember, we are talking about postural asphyxia which is asphyxia due to the position of the body and the position of the throat and the position of the tissues in the mouth and the position of the tongue. If we could bring a ripsaw in here and go through this man's head, I think you might be able to determine this, but unfortunately, such is not the case. This must be determined, in my opinion, and I am not sure it could even be determined in these circumstances, in all cases, how much postural asphyxia there really was for the simple reason that when a person dies all the muscles of the body relax and they may change position then.

In other words, even the tongue muscles relax when a person dies, and, so, consequently, the position of the tongue, when you examine the body, may not be exactly in the position it was in at the time this individual dies. And, therefore, I have to accept the reading and the research and the investigation that I have done with many of my colleagues who are in the field of anesthesiology and who have proven to me beyond a question of a doubt that people get into postural situations where they are unable to breathe because their airway is closed.

To finish my reasons, it seems to me that with the position of the body as we see it here in these pictures, that there is a logical assumption that there could have been postural asphyxiation in this case. In the absence of any other findings, and all the other things I know about the case, it seems to me that this is the most logical cause of death.

Q: Doctor, did you notice in the autopsy report or in any of the facts you had any evidence of pulmonary edema (effusion of fluid in the lungs)?

A: Well, he has no description of pulmonary edema. He says there is some congestion of the lungs anterior, but pulmonary edema as such I didn't read anything in the autopsy report about, no.

Q: What about the weight of the brain given in the autopsy report?

A: Well, as I remember, the weight of the brain was quite heavy. I will have to find that here. The brain weighed 1610 grams. This is certainly heavier than the usual adult brain as we see it at autopsy. I suppose this could be within the range of the upper limits of normal for brain weight, but actually the great majority of brains that I examine weigh somewhere between, oh, 1200 to 1400 grams, and this is a rather heavy weight, I would say, for a brain. Maybe he had a big head and a big brain. That is very possible.

Q: Does it have any significance to you or not insofar as your opinion as to the cause of death was concerned?

A: Yes. This indicates to me it is possible that this man had some degree of cerebral edema (effusion of fluid into the brain). I don't have any section of the brain to examine. I haven't any basis for making that statement except for the weight of the brain. I think I asked you to give me sections of the brain and you didn't have any to show me.

Q: Doctor, let me ask you now about the liver. I will ask you whether, based on the facts that you have before you, you have any opinion as to whether or not this man's death was caused by alcoholism?

A: Yes, I have an opinion about this, too.

Q: And what is that opinion?

A: Certainly nobody could exclude the possibility that this man was a chronic alcoholic and had died one of these sudden chronic alcoholic deaths, because I see them frequently and I would have to agree with many of the things Dr. Halpern has told you here this morning. I see unexplained deaths, and I see fatty livers in people, and to me, also, when you first showed me the section of this liver this possibility entered my mind that this man might be a chronic alcoholic and that maybe he did die one of these unexplained deaths.

I might add for the edification of the jury and also Your Honor that there has been much discovered even within the last three months about these sudden alcoholic deaths that we didn't know about even three months ago. There was a very recent presentation in Chicago at a national meeting of the Cardiovascular Society, a very excellent presentation bringing out new evidence of the cause of death in these sudden deaths of chronic alcoholics. This paper dealt with the electron microscopic changes which are present in heart muscle in persons who are chronic alcoholics and who were being treated for chronic alcoholism.

It has been demonstrated that in chronic alcoholics there are actual physical changes in the muscle of the heart, and also not only physical changes but also chemical changes. Now, this in itself may account for these sudden deaths that I see and that Dr. Halpern testified he sees in chronic alcoholics. Dr. Halpern told you that this is a flag or an indicator that a man might be a chronic alcoholic. I agree with this. I certainly thought of this when I first saw these pictures, but, again, this liver under the autopsy is described as a liver that weighs 1300 grams and showed no lesions. It says it is unremarkable except for moderate congestion.

Now, the normal weight of a liver of a man of Dr. Fry's size is approximately 1500 grams. In other words, this isn't even a big liver. This is a small liver. If anything, it is a couple of hundred grams smaller than the average weight of a liver for a man of this weight and size.

Now, when you have a fatty liver, a true fatty liver that I associate with chronic alcoholics, this liver is enlarged and heavy. It is enlarged because you have got a lot of fat in it. The sudden deaths that I have seen in chronic alcoholics who have had liver changes have been in most individuals who have had a great big liver that was just literally loaded with fat. There are many areas in this liver that I didn't think showed any severe degree of fatty metamorphosis or any degree of fatty infiltration, and this is not the usual type of liver I have associated with sudden, unexplainable deaths in alcoholics.

Another reason why I believe it is not a death from chronic alcoholism is that there are many, many conditions and diseases and abnormalities in a human body which can give you a liver that looks like this under the microscope besides chronic alcoholism.

To look at this and to show you some of my reasoning behind this, I might tell you the first hundred and fifty liver biopsies that were done in my community were done by myself, because when we first started doing liver biopsies, the surgeons were reluctant to do them. They were afraid they might run into the complications of hemorrhage and getting into bile ducts and causing the death of a patient, and for this reason and because of my anatomic knowledge of the liver I volunteered to do them. I wanted to do these biopsies on living human beings. Since that time I have examined many, many hundreds of liver biopsies which have been done by my colleagues, and I have seen livers like this in people who are ill from all kinds of reasons. I could make a photograph of those, and I would defy anybody to distinguish between those photographs and the photographs you have here in front of you.

So, to me this is not diagnostic of the assumption that this man was a chronic alcoholic.

Q. Doctor, let me ask you this. This condition here that you see, these fatty globules here, is this condition permanent or is it reversible, or can this condition be changed into what appears to be a healthy liver?

A. In my opinion this is a reversible condition. In other words, if what caused this fat to be in this liver, if the conditions which caused it, and I really don't know what caused this in this man, were reversed and he were put on a proper diet, proper vitamins, and the basic cause of this was removed, that this liver would revert to normal condition in a relatively short period of time. I have seen livers this badly infiltrated with fat, and we have had a second liver biopsy within a period of three days, and the liver will be perfectly normal.

Q. You heard Dr. Godwin testify a moment ago, a little while ago this morning that a diet deficiency could result in a fatty liver. Do you agree or disagree with that statement?

A. I agree with it completely. As a matter of fact, during World War II I was charged with investigating many of the prison camps in Europe, and we had severe cases of dietary deficiency of all types that we investigated in Dachau and in Landsburg, and many of the other prison camps, and pictures of livers like this were almost routine in these people who had severe dietary deficiencies. This type of a picture in the liver is not due to alcohol. This is not due to alcohol, in my opinion. This is due to other factors.

MR. HARMON:

Your witness.

MR. LOWE:

Q: Dr. Larson, as I understand it, you now devote a considerable amount of your time to the study of problems of how people died, is that correct?

A: Yes; I have for thirty years, sir.

Q: Yes, sir. And you have come here to Atlanta at the suggestion of counsel for the plaintiffs in this case to be a witness in the case, have you not?

A: That is correct. Mr. Harmon came to Tacoma and spent a day with me going over this case, and following that, I studied it for some time before I agreed to appear as a witness, sir.

Q: So, the answer to the exact question, that is, counsel asked you to come, is yes?

A: Yes, yes.

Q: All right, sir. And you have been here since when, last Friday?

A: No, sir. I arrived here Sunday night.

Q: Sunday night. And during the course of this trial you have been in the courtroom continuously, have you not?

A: Almost continuously, yes.

Q: And you have listened to the testimony given by all of the witnesses for the plaintiffs and for the defendants, have you not?

A: Yes, I have sir.

Q: Have you seen any other medical witness who has testified in the case who has been sitting in the courtroom during all of the giving of the evidence?

A: Would you explain what you mean by that, sir?

Q: Yes, sir. Have you seen any other doctor who has

identified himself as such and who has testified from the stand in the case who has sat here in the courtroom during all of the giving of the testimony?

A: Yes, I have seen several of them; yes, Mr. Lowe, I have.

Q: Well, Doctor, either you are not answering my question or you don't understand it, and I prefer to assume you don't understand it, because I am quite sure that one of us is under a misapprehension. Let me be direct. You saw Dr. Halpern while he was on the witness stand and heard him testify, did you not?

A: Yes, I did.

Q: Now, Dr. Halpern was not here listening while Dr. Godwin was testifying, was he?

A: No, sir.

Q: He was not in here listening while Dr. Dillon was testifying, was he?

A: No, sir.

Q: He was not in here listening while Dr. Steinhaus and Dr. Rumble were testifying, was he?

A: No, sir.

Q: And he was not in here while Dr. Adriani was testifying, was he?

A: That's correct.

Q: All right, sir. Now, the same thing is true with Dr. Dillon and Dr. Godwin, isn't it?

A: Yes, sir.

Q: So that you are the only doctor who has testified in the case who has sat throughout all of the testimony and listened to all of the testimony?

A: That is correct.

Q: You have said you prefer in all cases to go to the scene and see the body in an undisturbed position, correct?

A: That is correct, sir.

Q: In this case, of course, you did not have that privilege, did you?

A: No, I did not have that privilege.

Q: And you did not see the body at all?

A: No, I have never seen the body.

Q: Now, the things that you have learned about the condition of the body are things which you drew in part from the report of Dr. Dillon, is that correct?

A: That is correct, yes.

Q: And you have outlined certain other things in your earlier testimony that you considered and studied, have you not?

A: That is correct.

Q: All right, sir. Doctor, you have made a comment about the mark on the left cheek as shown in at least two of the photographs which have been many times identified here. Isn't it correct that ordinarily when there is a bruise caused by a substantial blow that one of the results is a swelling?

A: That is true. It depends on the length of time the deceased lived as to how much swelling there will be, yes. In other words, in an individual who died rather rapidly there would be little time for much swelling to develop because the circulation would have ceased.

Q: But the answer to the precise question I asked you is yes, as you gave it?

A: Yes. I said if there was a sufficient amount of time for the swelling to occur.

Q: I understand, yes, sir. Now, Doctor, the question as to the effect of an outer force upon the body depends upon how that force is applied and the quantity of that force, doesn't it?

A: Yes, sir. Certainly those are two of the factors that you will take into consideration, yes.

Q: Now, one of the things that happens sometimes when a force is applied to the cheekbone of the body is that the cheekbone may break, isn't that right?

A: This is somewhat unusual in my experience, but it may happen.

Q: It can happen?

A: It can happen, yes.

Q: One thing which occurs when a force is applied to the body, if the force is applied to the skull, that is, the bony part of the skull, is that the skull may break, cause a skull fracture, isn't that so?

A: Certainly this does happen, yes.

Q: One of the things that occurs when there is a substantial blow to the head, or at least to the upper part of the head, is that even though there might not be a bone fracture there may very well be findings on or in the brain to illustrate the fact that force was applied, isn't that correct?

A: Yes. This is one reason we do autopsies, sir.

Q: When we find that there is nothing shown in the brain, then we are able to make a conclusion that the force applied was not sufficient to make a showing on or in the brain, isn't that right?

A: Would you repeat that question?

Q: Yes, sir. When we find that there is nothing shown on or in the brain, then we are able to conclude that the force was not sufficient to cause anything to be shown on or in the brain?

A: I think the answer to that would be obvious, yes, sir.

Q: You understand, Doctor, I am asking you some rather, perhaps, rather basic questions?

A: Yes, sir.

Q: While you feel that it might have been better to take a piece of the tissue out of the marked area on the left cheek and preserve it for microscopic study, had you been examining this body, you are not able, since you did not see the body, to tell whether you would have determined to do that or not, is that correct?

A: Well, my answer to that, Mr. Lowe, would be that in all cases of this kind, even though there is a lesion on the face where you don't wish to disfigure anyone I would have taken a section of this. This is my routine procedure.

Q: Doctor, I am being pretty basic now, and I am being this basic. Since you weren't there and didn't participate in the examination of the body after death, what you are saying to this jury is what you believe you would have done, but since you didn't do it you don't know whether you would have done it or not?

A: No, I would have—

Q: Isn't that right?

A: Yes, I would have to answer that yes.

Q: What one does, in connection with a problem, depends on how the problem presents itself, is this not so?

A: Well, I think this is a very fair statement, yes, sir.

Q: I will put it this way: If a person is presented with a problem and if the person does the best he can do or feels that he can do under the circumstances, then he has done the best he can or feels he can do under those circumstances, but if later hindsight illustrates something to the contrary, this is an unfortunate thing in life, isn't it?

A: Yes, it is, sir.

Q: We are not all perfect, are we?

A: No, we are not; above all, not me.

Q: This applies to all of us who are human, doesn't it? Now, Doctor, you spoke of the weight of the brain reflected in the autopsy report and you accepted that weight as being correct, didn't you?

A: Yes. Remembered the weight at 1610 grams out of the autopsy report.

Q: Yes. And this weight is an indication of a brain that is somewhat heavier than normal, isn't it?

A: I think I made the statement, Mr. Lowe, that this is heavier than the usual average brains that I have weighed at the time of autopsy.

Q: The liver slide which you saw is a slide that does give reasonable indication to a doctor that this person might have been an alcoholic, correct?

A: No, I don't think that is correct, Mr. Lowe. I would say that to those few of us who specialize in this field and are cognizant of what alcohol can do, I think the real specialist in this field would recognize that as an indication that could mean this person was a chronic alcoholic, although I have had a great deal of trouble selling this to my colleagues even in pathology.

Q: Yes, sir. But it seems to have been accepted by you and Dr. Halpern and by Dr. Godwin?

A: Oh, yes.

Q: All right, sir.

A: Yes.

Q: I believe that you referred to the phrase "dietary deficiency," and I believe you also heard Dr. Godwin make some reference to the phrase "dietary deficiency," or some similar phrase, correct?

A: Yes, sir.

Q: The dietary deficiency that is indicated by this sort of liver—let me rephrase it. As to the dietary deficiency indicated by this sort of liver, we have again a flag or a clue to indicate that there may have been a dietary deficiency, isn't that so?

A: Yes, Mr. Lowe. In my opinion what we see in this liver, the primary factor, is, in my opinion, in most instances, a liver like this would be due to certain dietary deficiency and not due to the alcohol itself. I don't think the alcohol caused this at all.

Q: The dietary deficiency is an indicator that the person has not been taking in food properly and has not been making proper use of food, isn't that right?

A: It could be either one or both.

Q: Or a combination of the two?

A: Yes.

Q: Yes, sir. And a person who has gotten into a condition of this kind can come fairly quickly to a terminal or death condition, can he not?

A: I think I answered that this morning by saying that in my experience the ones who are alcoholics that I have been able to get a good history of had a liver that was much larger than this and much more seriously infiltrated with fat than I see in this particular liver here, but I suppose my answer to your question would have to be yes, it could happen in a person with a liver that looked like this. Is that what you are asking?

Q: Yes, sir.

A: Yes, sir, my answer would be yes.

Q: Doctor, you, of course, do not know when the mark on the left side of the cheek of Dr. Fry literally was made, do you? You weren't there and didn't see it?

A: No, I do not know how it was made.

Q: All right, sir. What you would say about this, then, is a deduction on your part, isn't it?

A: I would say it is a deduction, yes. Based on what evidence I have available to me.

Q: Yes, sir. And what you do is take whatever evidence is available to you and think about it and come up with a conclusion as to a possibility or a series of possibilites, isn't that right?

A: That is correct.

Q: And one of the possibilities that we see here is that the bruise might have been made when the person came to the floor, isn't it?

A: Oh, yes. I thought of this. I put this under the microscope, with the possibility in mind that I could see some evidence of a cross-hatch mark in this.

Q: Which would indicate the sort of mark that you would expect from the weave of the rug as shown in other photographs?

A: I don't know the weave of the rug, but under the microscope, Mr. Lowe, the front part of this wound here does show a pattern which very well could be due to a rug. I don't know this of my own knowledge, but it certainly could be so.

Q: All right, sir. So that you feel that one of the reasonable possibilities is that the pattern portion of that mark could have come from the rug on the floor?

A: Oh, yes, I should say so.

Q: Now, Doctor, a person who suffers from convulsions will sometimes find that his body is temporarily not subject to complete control, isn't that right?

A: Yes. I think in a generalized convulsion you can say that the individual has no control of his body.

Q: All right. So we start with that as a premise. Now, if Dr. Fry had a generalized convulsion as a result of a dietary deficiency or as a result of an alcoholic condition, he might well have gone to the floor without any control over his physical body, isn't that so?

A: You would certainly have to say this, yes.

Q: Yes, sir. And he could have come to rest on the floor on his left cheek as well as on any other part of the body?

A: Oh, yes, most certainly.

Q: And he could have ended up with his arms in the position illustrated but not completely shown by the pictures, couldn't he?

A: Yes. As a matter of fact, I feel from the pictures he really didn't have consciousness when he fell, because it is a natural thing to put your arms out, Mr. Lowe, when you fall. This isn't invariably true, but it certainly is the natural thing for a person to do. I have seen falls where people did not do this, but, on the other hand, this is the ordinary thing for a person to do.

Q: Yes, sir. So if we take the ordinary thing, so far as a fall is concerned, then we would presume he would put his hands in some other position?

A: I think this would be the ordinary thing to do.

Q: Yes. And then if we say that this was not ordinary because his arms did not appear to have been put out that way, then we have to conclude that he came down either because he was in a seizure of a physical discomfort or because something else had happened to him rendering him unconscious while he was on the way down, don't we?

A: I certainly think this is a possibility, yes.

Q: And this is the most likely possibility, that is, that he was unconscious on the way down, isn't it?

A: I think so, yes.

MR. LOWE:

"That's all, Your Honor."

REDIRECT EXAMINATION

MR. HARMON:

Q: Doctor, assume a man is knocked unconscious by a blow. Would this blow be reflected in actual damage that you could see on the brain?

A: Well, I would say in the great majority of the cases where a person is knocked unconscious by a blow, that there would not be anything a pathologist or anybody else could see in the brain or inside the head. Take boxing matches, for example, I have examined the brains of a large number of boxers who have been knocked out on many occasions, and examination of their brains after they die will disclose absolutely nothing. I think it is a matter of common knowledge you can be knocked out and not have a brain hemorrhage or brain lesion that you could discover at autopsy. The term that is used to describe this is a concussion of the brain. In other words, if you get hit on the side of the head, it shakes the brain. The brain is in a little fluid package inside the head in which it has a chance to move from one side to the other.

If you get a blow to one side of the head, the brain will move in this fluid compartment, and this will disturb the nerve cells sufficiently so that you lose consciousness. If you are unfortunate enough to tear a blood vessel when you do this, then you will have a hemorrhage. But certainly most of the people who get rendered unconscious by, say, a blow fortunately don't have anything you can see in the brain, or many of us wouldn't be here today.

Q: Now, did you take the fact into consideration that, as you testified to Mr. Lowe a minute or two ago, that there was a possibility that Dr. Fry was not fully conscious at the time that he hit the floor, did you take that fact into consideration with the other facts that we gave you this morning when you reached your opinion that you did as to the cause of his death?

A: Oh, yes.

Q: No further questions.

RECROSS-EXAMINATION

MR. LOWE:

Q: Doctor, where you have a situation where it is contended that a blow caused unconsciousness and you find nothing in the brain, that is, in the examination of the brain after death, all you can really say is that you have found nothing in the brain, but if there was a blow, unconsciousness is one of the possibilities, isn't it?

A: Yes. I based my opinion, Mr. Lowe, as to the fact that this man was unconscious by the fact of the way his body was found.

Q: Well, let me suggest this to you—it may not be sensible, but there are some marks on my head made in various ways not material here. Isn't it possible that some of the marks on my head which may have caused various injuries could have been made and I not become unconscious?

A: Oh, yes, yes.

Q: Now, a lot of marks, cuts and bruises made on the head don't cause unconsciousness?

A: That is correct, sir.

Q: So the fact that a mark exists does not mean that there was any unconsciousness just because a mark is there?

A: Not because of the mark itself, no.

Q: All right, sir. Now, if the mark is bad enough to cause unconsciousness, we can be sure that it did within reason do damage to the brain, can't we?

A: Not necessarily. This is a hobby of mine, Mr. Lowe. I used to be a boxer, and I have been affiliated with the boxing business since youth. I have seen cases of boxers, for example, who have had rather severe intracranial injuries who have gotten up and answered a bell and went on fighting. So I don't think I could answer your question "yes." My answer would have to be "no."

Q: But it is pretty good evidence, isn't it?

A: It is good evidence, yes.

Q: That is all, Doctor.

It was about all, at that—except for a wire Dr. Larson received a few hours after he returned to Tacoma. "DR. CHARLES P. LARSON, TACOMA GENERAL HOSPITAL, TACOMA, WASHINGTON: WE WON, THANKS TO YOUR GOOD EFFORTS, LETTER FOLLOWS... HARMON."

It wasn't necessary to add that with the victory went $1,000,000 to the Fry family, but in subsequent appeals this figure was reduced somewhat.

Oh Lordy, how sweet it was. It called for a celebration, and that night Dr. Larson celebrated like it was the first day of the world.

Alcoholics, Inc.

THE writer sipped his tea and listened.

"Alcohol affects all five senses of the human body," said the doctor, wiping his mouth with the napkin. "Do you know what they are?"

"Let's see," the writer said. "There's vision, hearing, taste, and touch. What's the fifth?"

"Olfactory—the sense of smell," replied the doctor.

"Smell?"

"Yes. Booze depresses it. Get a person drunk enough and he may not even detect the passing of gas."

"You mean," the writer asked, putting it crudely, "if I fart, he won't even smell it?"

"Exactly," the doctor said. "The principal effect of alcohol on our bodies is on the nerve cells. It always produces a neurological depression which is probably due to an interference of oxidation within nerve cells. The degree of depression is not linear, since twice as much alcohol does not produce twice as much neurological depression but an exponential increase which is much more than double the effect."

"On the other hand, alcohol serves as a social stimulant."

"Yes," the doctor said. "It takes a variety of forms and varies to a degree which bears no constant relation to the amount of drink a person consumes. Reactions vary from hysterical gaiety to 'crying in your beer.' Some people begin to swing from the chandeliers after only a few drinks, while others steadily and calmly go at it drink after drink with little outward effect until they fall flat on their face."

"Why the difference?" the writer wanted to know.

"A number of factors are involved," the doctor said. "Environment, mental attitude, personality—they all play a role in determining how a person reacts to liquor. The apparent stimulation of individuals under the influence of alcohol is due to a release of the higher brain centers, leading to euphoria and spontaneity."

"Does liquor affect a man's resistance to hypoxia?" the writer asked.

"What do you know about hypoxia?"

"I looked it up."

"And?"

"It means a deficiency of oxygen reaching the tissues of the body."

"To answer your question, then; yes, alcohol *significantly* reduces a person's resistance to the effects of hypoxia. This makes liquor hazardous to mountain climbers, aviators and anyone who has a cardiac or pulmonary condition with borderline hypoxia."

"What about the other four senses? Vision, for example?"

"Tests have demonstrated that with increasing amounts of alcohol, the acuity progressively diminishes to the point where vision is obscured to a level comparable to wearing dark sunglasses at night. Driving a car with 150 mg of blood alcohol might be compared to a person wearing dark sunglasses at night with a pair of binoculars strapped in front of the eyes. At higher levels, somewhere between 100 to 200 mg, ocular coordination is objectively impaired and diplopia appears."

"Diplopia?"

"Double vision. The driver sees two, four or eight lines in the center lane instead of the normal single line. The driver may close one eye so that he can keep the single line on the road in focus. His vision may then be compared to that of a man wearing sunglasses at night having a telescope strapped over the open eye."

"I've heard it said," the writer remarked, "that too much booze dims an individual's hearing. True?"

The doctor nodded.

"Yes," he said. "To prove this, you only need to observe the loudness of conversation as a cocktail party progresses. After most of the guests have had three or four drinks, someone arriving late, cold sober, would compare the sound to that of the loud buzzing of a beehive. People tend to talk louder as the party and the alcohol level increases. This also explains why so many people fail to hear the sound of horns or train whistles when drunk."

"How does liquor affect the sense of touch?"

"The drunker one gets, the more it diminishes. This is probably the origin of the old saying, 'He is in no pain.' There's a diminished sensation to pain not unlike that from other anesthetics. This accounts for the frequent cigarette burns on the hands of chronic alcoholics."

"Does alcohol have much the same effect on taste?"

"Very much so. The sense of taste lessens in accordance to how much you drink. In a pleasant state of inebriation all food tastes good. This is probably the reason why cocktails are always served at parties prior to the meal. We have all attended perfectly 'dry' banquets in which, although the food was excellently prepared, it did not please all the guests. I'm sure if alcohol had been served before the meal, there'd have been no complaints even if the quality of the food was poor. I have personally seen people who will drink only one kind of whiskey, but after a drink or two it is possible to switch brands on them without so much as a peep."

About 30 years ago, Dr. Larson became involved in a study on alcoholism. Today he is an internationally recognized authority on the subject. He has served on The Committee of Alcohol and Drugs of the National Safety Council for three decades. He has written numerous papers on alcoholism, including a popular chapter ("Alcohol: Fact and Fallacy") in a medical-legal book *(Legal Medicine Annual 1969,* edited by Cyril H. Wecht, Appleton-Century-Crofts, New York) which is still selling after nine years. Dr. Larson has also lectured extensively from coast to coast on alcoholism.

To put it bluntly, we are at war on the home front against the disease. The police are the front line, and over the years, Dr. Larson has been right up there with them.

Dr. Larson

> Approximately 55,000 people are killed in the United States each year by automobile accidents; 1,700,000 are injured. This represents *billions* of dollars a year expense.
>
> Much of the problem is due to alcohol.
>
> Recent surveys indicate that in over 50 percent of the one-car fatalities, the driver of the automobile had been drinking. In over 75 percent of the cases where there is a two-car accident which is fatal, one or the other of the drivers was drunk. My own statistics indicate that in over 60 percent of all fatal pedestrian accidents either the driver of the car or the pedestrian was intoxicated. More recently, the incidence of the use of alcohol in private airplane pilots involved in accidents has been alarmingly high, even up to 75 percent.
>
> The National Safety Council has estimated that an individual with a blood alcohol level of 150 mg is 55 times as likely to become involved in an accident, and that at 100 mg he is 15 times as likely compared to a sober driver. Sociological studies indicate that a large group of the so-

called drunken drivers are comprised of those who are chronic alcoholics.

It is a common fallacy that drinking coffee will sober up a person. Only time will produce a sobering effect. Stressful incidents, such as accidents, arrest by an officer or emotional shock, may lead to temporary improvement of the objective signs of drunkenness, but even under these conditions the average person will revert to the same degree or objective impairment in a matter of minutes.

Judgment is one of the first mental functions affected by alcohol. This blunting of judgment is often the factor which leads to automobile accidents, poor business decisions, gambling losses, fights and injuries.

The faculty of attention deteriorates rapidly with the use of alcohol. This is undoubtedly one of the principal reasons why individuals even with low levels of alcohol end up as traffic victims.

Ability to learn is blunted by the use of alcohol. This is attested to by such common knowledge as the inability to recall anything about what a lecturer said after a dinner preceded by cocktails except that it was a "fine speech." Recall memory is often markedly disturbed by relatively small amounts of alcohol in which individuals cannot accurately recall certain situations or even names of people whom they have known for years.

Motor skills are also retarded. It has been proven times without number that the reaction time of individuals becomes impaired at relatively low levels of blood alcohol. It is common knowledge that skill in the performance of various athletic activities and games involving precision deteriorates with increasing amounts of blood alcohol. Expert golfers, bowlers, horseshoe pitchers or dartsmen can readily attest to the deterioration of their skills when they drink too much.

Alcohol also affects the emotions. It has been called the great leveler and in a sense acts as a tranquilizer for many people.

It is generally believed that moral standards are blunted and lowered by the use of alcohol. Liquor can quickly seduce and expand our egos. Impulse becomes master as restraint blows out, and all barriers—legal, moral and social—melt away. Alcohol partially narcotizes the nerve centers, leading to the propensity to distort reality, producing an irresistible sexual image of ourselves. We are full of ideas, a good many of them carnal, and it is a waste of time trying to convince anyone at such moments that liquor is not a true aphrodisiac. This leads to the bar-and-brothel combination, sex offenses, illegitimacy and lessened ability of the intoxicated to take proper prophylactic and contraceptive precautions. Fundamentally, however, the point to keep in mind is the similarity between drinking as such, and sexual activity as such. Alcohol increases the desire for sex but markedly impairs the performance; prolonged intercourse without ejaculation is often the result. Alcohol unabashes action, drowns the conscience and murders fastidiousness. Enough booze can make you see a whore as a Mona Lisa. Sample:

Maisie was a London whore on Piccadilly Square. She picked up a drunk and took him to her bedroom where he died during the act. Appearing in court the next morning, the judge asked her: "Maisie, please tell the court exactly what happened."

"Well, your Honor," she said, "I thought he was a-comin', but he really was a-goin.'"

Alcoholism has been called the No. 1 public health enemy. It has been estimated that there are some 6.5 million male alcoholics in the U.S. Indirectly this disease affects 25 to 30 million other people. Many deaths and diseases are directly attributable to liquor. It is the most common poison known to man.

One of the most dramatic deaths not infrequently witnessed by forensic pathologists is that of the youngster who on a dare drinks a large amount (6 to 10 ounces) of whiskey on an empty stomach and dies as a result of a high temporary blood alcohol level. Various studies indicate that from 25 to 50 percent of all suicides involve individuals under the influence of alcohol. For homicide the rate is between 50 and 60 percent. There are thousands of statistics relating alcohol to crime. Anyone performing medico-legal autopsies is familiar with the high incidence of intoxication in both the victim and the murderer. It has been estimated that between 50 and 70 percent of all felons, including those engaged in burglary, armed robbery, theft, forgery, shoplifting, etc., have a high incidence rate of intoxication or alcohol imbibition prior to committing the crime.

One of the most common causes of death in alcoholics is an undiagnosed and untreated pneumonia. Alcohol in the tracheobronchial tree is a well-proven irritant. This can be the direct cause of the undiagnosed pneumonia in the alcoholic.

"Traumatic deaths are extremely common in alcoholics," Dr. Larson states. "Cerebral trauma with its complications is the commonest cause of death in alcoholics. I have frequently observed a ruptured spleen with massive intra-abdominal hemorrhage as the cause of death in an alcoholic which resulted from abdominal trauma which the deceased disregarded. Fights involving a customer and a bartender frequently result in fatal trauma to the alcoholic.

"Approximately 30 percent of all individuals dying from accidental burns have either been drunk or were burned because someone else was drunk. Booze and carbon monoxide do not mix. It is my opinion that an individual who has had too much to drink will die at a much lower carbon monoxide concentration than will a sober person. This is probably due to the hypoxic effect of the alcohol added to the hypoxic effect of the carbon monoxide. This is often seen in lover's lane or motel deaths when the intoxicated person will be found dead from carbon monoxide and alcohol, whereas the sober individual will survive."

A high percentage of exposure deaths (in some surveys, up to 65 percent) are associated with drinking. All drowning victims should have a blood alcohol determination, because in a high percentage of cases the alcohol level will be moderately or severely elevated. The same is true in scuba diving deaths.

Both malnutrition and obesity are frequently associated with chronic alcoholism. Severe fatty infiltration of the heart has been observed in alcoholics.

Many studies have been made on the rate of metabolism of alcohol in the human body. These studies indicate that humans metabolize alcohol at a rate varying between 12 and 20 mg per 100 ml of blood per hour. The average is probably in the neighborhood of 15 to 17 mg per hour in a normal person. This means that the average drinker will burn up approximately one ounce of *absolute* alcohol every three hours. For purposes of rough calculation, it is easier to visualize that the average individual will burn one ounce of 85 proof bar whiskey or one 12-ounce bottle of beer per hour. The average person can only consume and metabolize about one fifth (26 ounces) of whiskey per day. There are exceptional individuals who can metabolize alcohol faster. On the other hand, many chronic alcoholics develop liver damage and consequently their rate of alcohol metabolism is markedly depressed so that a few ordinary drinks will keep them drunk for hours.

"In most people, it is generally believed that just a few drinks will bring the blood alcohol level up to 100 mg. Such is not the case. Years ago, prior to our present knowledge of how many drinks are required to reach the 100 mg blood level, my own attorney and I conducted a series of personal experiments on ourselves," Dr. Larson recalls. "Once a week for several weeks we would meet in my office after work, divide and consume a pint (16 ounces) of 86-proof bourbon on an empty stomach in a period of less than an hour. A standby medical technologist drew our blood at stipulated intervals. At no time did either of us reach the 100 mg level, although on occasion one or the other of us would have levels in the 90s. We both agreed that neither of us was physically nor psychologically capable of safely driving an automobile. We also discovered that loading our stomachs with carbohydrates prior to drinking and by using straight whiskey instead of diluted whiskey, we could consume approximately *twice* as much with *half* the effect. So if I were to advise someone how to drink another man 'under the table,' I would tell him to load up on food, particularly proteins and carbohydrates, drink nothing but straight whiskey, indulge only in *serious* conversations and control his emotions. Under these circumstances he could consume an inordinate amount of whiskey and still be relatively in command of his faculties and on his feet. However, eventually the alcohol would become diluted and absorbed, and the piper would be paid."

There is much dispute in the medical literature regarding the relationship between alcohol and cancer. Some reports have indicated an increased incidence of mouth, esophageal and liver cancer in chronic alcoholics. Statistically it is difficult to prove this association because most chronic alcoholics do not live much beyond the age of 50 and, consequently, have not reached the cancer age. Due to the premature deaths of most alcoholics, it is impossible to obtain valid statistics on the incidence of arteriosclerosis, stroke and many other geriatric diseases in chronic alcoholics. In the past alcohol has been prescribed by some physicians to prevent heart disease. There is no valid evidence that alcohol prevents arteriosclerosis. Certainly alcohol diminishes the coronary flow and increases the load on the heart.

Alcoholism is in itself a form of chronic suicide. Some individuals can actually commit suicide by excessive alcohol ingestion per se, provided they do not develop pylorospasm and vomit.

It's a hell of a way to go.

The Bird That Killed Like a Hawk

I was a reporter, a John-of-all-trades, for the old *Tacoma Times* at the time. I had come to the city's No. 2 newspaper in 1947 under the sponsorship of Elliot Metcalf to do sports. I did them—but not on Thursdays. Because we had a very small staff, on the fourth day of the week I was "loaned" to the city editor, Paul Busselle, to be available for handyman service.

On October 30, 1947, I was working obituaries. That is, I'd call up the various mortuaries around town, find out who'd died in the last 24 hours and then say something nice about the departed for the afternoon editions. I hated dead Thursdays. It was not exactly the most inspiring journalism for a 23-year-old with uncorked vigor. It gave me the creeps.

Paul Busselle was a modest city editor, respected for his professionalism and admired for his fairness. At the same time he was a taskmaster and demanded absolute perfection. Upon his round, austere face stood an ample nose, like a blob of putty and a weather vane of his moods. Its chief attribute was its ability to change expression. A well-written story found his nostrils dilated, as if smelling flowers. A poor job of reporting brought severe lines to his face, like a fallen frown.

Late that morning, Busselle got the news. There had been a sensational double murder up on South J Street and the *Tacoma News Tribune* had it splashed all over the front page:

> NEGRO CAUGHT OUTSIDE HOME BY POLICE
>
> A mother and her 17-year-old daughter were dead, two policemen were wounded and a 45-year-old Negro was in jail facing murder charges this Thursday morning after a night of horror whose pattern of attempted rape and bludgeoning police officers spent the night attempting to piece together.
>
> The dead are Mrs. Bertha Kludt, 52, a widow, and Miss Beverly June Kludt, beautiful brunette graduate of Lincoln High School, class of 1947.
>
> Officers Andres P. Sabutis and Evan Davies were knifed in the capture of burly Jake Bird, transient who is said to have admitted the slayings . . .

Bussell's face turned a million shades of red when he saw the Trib story. We'd been completely scooped. Our first edition carried no mention of the murders.

"All right," Paul snapped. "We still have the late afternoon edition. You—McCallum; you—Herbert. Get down to the police station and see if there's anything new on the story."

Frank Herbert was the paper's photographer-reporter; a crackerjack staff man. He is the same Frank Herbert who, today, is one of the world's leading science-fiction novelists (*Dune*, with 10 million sales world-wide, The *Dosadi Experiment*, etc.). He grabbed his camera and, together, we bolted down the stairs and out the door.

Outside, the rain beat with the persistence of an unpaid madam. A small wind carried random snorts of pellets, puddling the streets. The rain made a gutter of my hatbrim. It trickled inside the collar of my raincoat as we raced for the station house, two blocks down 11th Street hill and several more blocks north on Pacific. I swore at the weather as we sloshed past the newsstand on Broadway and heard the newsboy hawking the Trib: "EXTRA! EXTRA! MURDER CHARGES FILED IN DOUBLE SLAYINGS. READ ALL ABOUT IT. GET YOUR PAPER." Damn that Bill Dugovich. Bill covered the police beat for the *News Tribune* like a jealous bulldog. He was a great reporter—very competitive. In those days the *Times* and the *News Tribune* had a hot rivalry going.

At the jailhouse Jake Bird was under tight security. When Frank sought permission to take some pictures of him, he was told no. "No one goes near the prisoner," an officer said. "He's too dangerous, we don't want you gettin' hurt."

Frank was persistent, however, and he finally talked one of the officers into giving him five minutes outside Bird's cell. He'd take the pictures, he said, through the bars.

Inside security, Frank was ushered along to Bird's isolation cell. Through the bars was revealed a black, bald fellow, six-feet, 185 pounds, who looked like he'd just come out of a street brawl with the devil himself. There was a hole in the top of his nose, the skin around his eyes and cheeks was puffed up like he'd just tangled with a nest of hornets, and his clothes were splattered with dry blood stains. He was a mess. He lay like a dissected frog on the iron bed.

Frank remembers asking Bird, "Do you mind if I take a couple of pictures? I'm from the *Times*."

Bird lifted himself to his feet, sucked in his breath, blinked—and posed. When he smiled, there was a big gap in his broken front teeth.

"I feel like a beaten elephant after the kill," Bird said.

"What did you do to deserve this?" Frank wanted to know.

"I did nothing," Bird said. "They got the wrong fellow." It was to become one of Jake Bird's favorite lines.

Meanwhile, I went after Patrolman Skip Davies, one of the two officers who nailed Bird. He was a mountain of a man with a man's-man figure; six-feet-three; 250 pounds. A regular big buster of a fellow—wrestler's muscles, broad shoulders and a thin, black mustache on a long-jawed, confident face. Yes, he said, he was one of the arresting officers. Calmly, he recounted the details.

"Officer Tiny Sabutis and I had been sitting in our patrol wagon in front of Smitty's Drive-In, down on Puyallup Avenue, listening to the police dispatcher. The radio never let up. With all ears we listened. Suddenly: 'There's a woman screaming in the neighborhood of the 2000 block on South J Street!' I said to Tiny, 'That's us!' and he rolled the car. We were approximately 20 blocks away and, floorboarding it, were there within five minutes. We pulled up in front of 2018 South J Street, where a Mrs. Steinsiefer was waiting for us. She said she had heard screaming. It came, she said, from the house around the corner. Tiny went to the back door and I went to the front. I no sooner hit the front porch when Tiny shouted, 'Skip, watch out. There's a man running around the side of the house—and he's got something in his hand!'"

Neither Davies nor Sabutis yet knew, of course, what the story was inside the house, and as the fleeing man swept past him on the dead run, Davies, a former football tackle, took off after him. He chased him for a block and a half over backyard fences. Whatever the suspect was carrying in his hand, he lost it while vaulting the first fence he came to.

Finally, at 2122 South J, Officer Davies cornered him. It was a very black night, drizzling, and 2:20 a.m. Davies pulled his revolver. The suspect was hidden behind bushes in the backyard.

"Show yourself or I'll shoot," Davies commanded. Suddenly, from out of the dark, the man rushed Officer Davies. Davies turned and swung his pistol, smashing the suspect flush on the face. Fiercely—instinctively—the attacker fought back like a madman. He was screaming curses at the top of his lungs and giving way to personal animosity, to hysteria—to all those animal reactions that are demonstrated in hand-to-hand combat. The man had a knife now and slashed at Davies with it, cutting him on the hand. While in this desperate squeeze, Davies shouted for Sabutis and then clubbed the man to the ground with his pistol. The man had the strength of a bucking horse. When Sabutis arrived and leaned over him to put the handcuffs on him, the wielder cut him up the back, leaving a five-inch gash. The sight of all that blood infuriated Officer Davies. Avoiding a kick aimed at his groin, he socked back once, twice, three times with firmly planted punches. The suspect's face bled like a cut tomato under the impact of Officer Davies' 250 hysterical pounds. When it was all over, the suspect lay on the ground, panting.

Dumbly, Officer Davies looked down at the man at his feet. There was blood oozing slowly down the scalp and nose and dripping from his chin in bright drops. In a spasm of blind hatred, Davies yelled at him, "You dirty sonofabitch! Try to kill me, will you! Nobody can pull that stuff on *me*!"

Eight hours later, his hands were still shaking.

All three men required attention at the hospital. The police officers were treated at St. Joseph's, the suspect at the County Hospital. The five-inch gash in Sabutis' back kept him in the hospital for several days, but his partner, Davies, with no more damage than a bandaged hand, felt healthy enough to go with Officer Paul Gookins back to the death scene.

Officer Skip Davies:

> Because it was still dark, we got some high-powered lights and backtracked the course in which Sabutis and I had chased the suspect. In the rear of 1010 South 21st Street, we found both his shoes, which of all things, he'd been carrying while I chased him. We also found an iron sashweight in the backyard of 2112 South J. As that was the course he took, he possibly had the sashweight in his

> possession, so we took that in evidence too. Then we went into the house—for the first time—and found the victims: Beverly Kludt, 22, and Bertha Kludt, 52, her mother. Their neighbors thought very highly of them. They were well-liked. Beverly's body was lying on the floor in a small dining nook between the kitchen and the passage to the bedrooms. Her mother was lying in one of the bedrooms. Both had been beaten with the blunt nose and cut with the blade of an axe. Both were dead, clothed in disarranged nightgowns; there were signs of a fierce struggle around both women. Blood was spattered everywhere. Officer Gookins and I then put in a call to homicide and remained at the scene, to secure it against unauthorized persons, and until photographs had been taken, diagrams made and the bodies removed.

The suspect had put up such resistance that he had to be forcibly subdued, both by Patrolman Davies and by authorities at the County Hospital. As frantic resistance can be an indication of guilt, the Tacoma Police started a "make" on the suspect—now identified as Jake Bird, Black, Male—and before the night was out answers and queries began to come in on him.

Before the flood crested, the implications of Jake Bird's involvement in similar crimes previous to the killings of the two Kludt women built up as follows:

The Houston, Texas, Police Department wanted him questioned in respect to the murder of Mrs. Harry L. Richardson. The Chicago Police Department was interested in a weighted body dumped into Lake Michigan about five miles south of Kenosha. The Los Angeles Police Department asked for clarification of a murder of a "Jewish grocer" on General Avenue and of a young colored by by the name of "Lively." The New York City Police Department had a delicatessen robbery and the murder of the owner that pointed to Bird.

Dr. Charles Larson was a colonel in the U.S. Army Medical Corps in Germany during WW II. The Mercedes-Benz was "traded" (under orders from the commanding general of the 7th Army) for a red Mercedes convertible. The 16-cylinder special, one of only three cars built, was a gift from a grateful German to Col. Larson for attending a daughter. The general later killed himself when the car ran off a winding mountain highway.

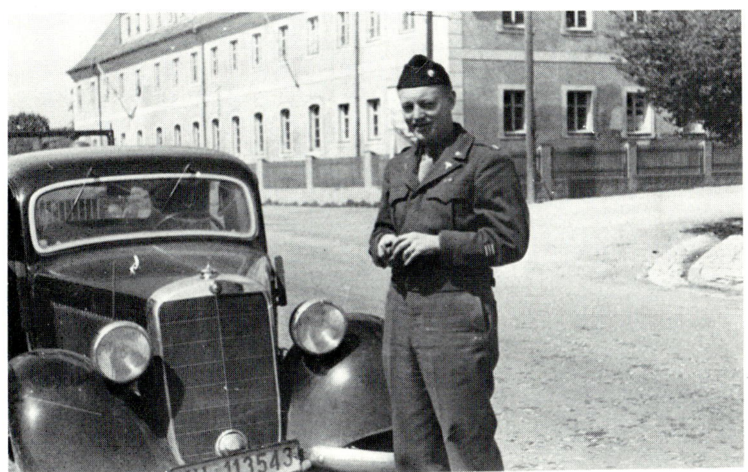

As the only forensic pathologist on duty in the southern German theater, Col. Larson entered Dachau only hours after it was liberated to find stacks of bodies. This photo taken by Dr. Larson displayed the horrendous scenes at the death camp. Dr. Larson performed more than a thousand autopsies at Dachau.

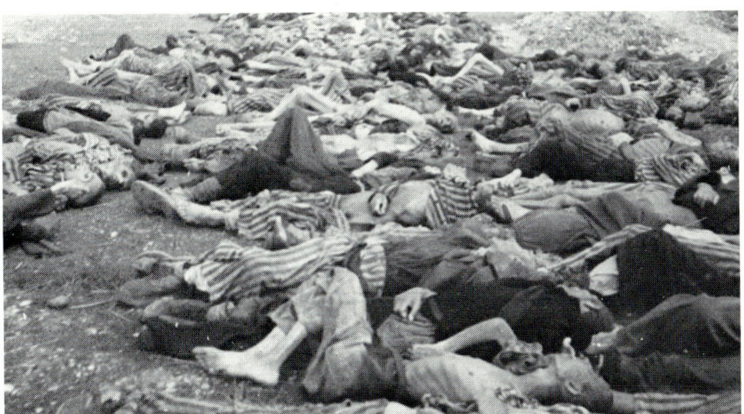

Major General Freeman pinned the U.S. Army Medal of Commendation on Col. Charles Larson in 1965.

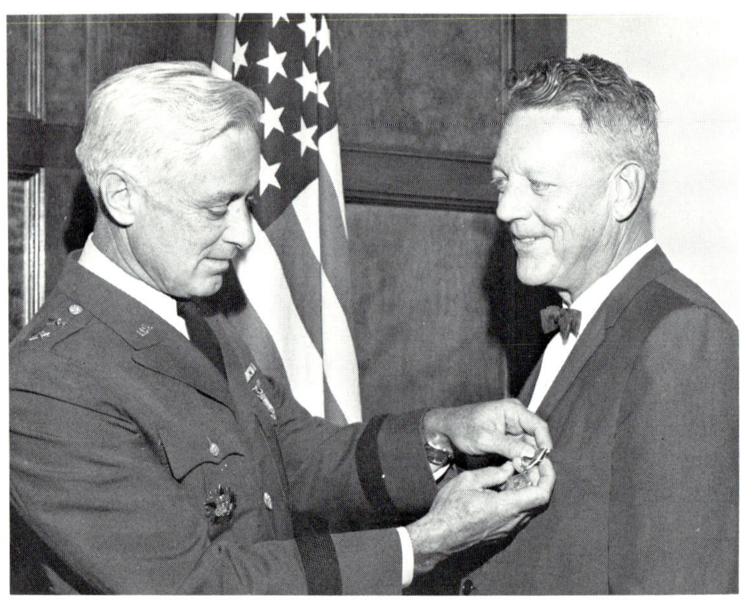

In 1964 Col. Larson turned over his command of the 359th Reserve General Hospital to Lt. Col. Clinton A. Piper.

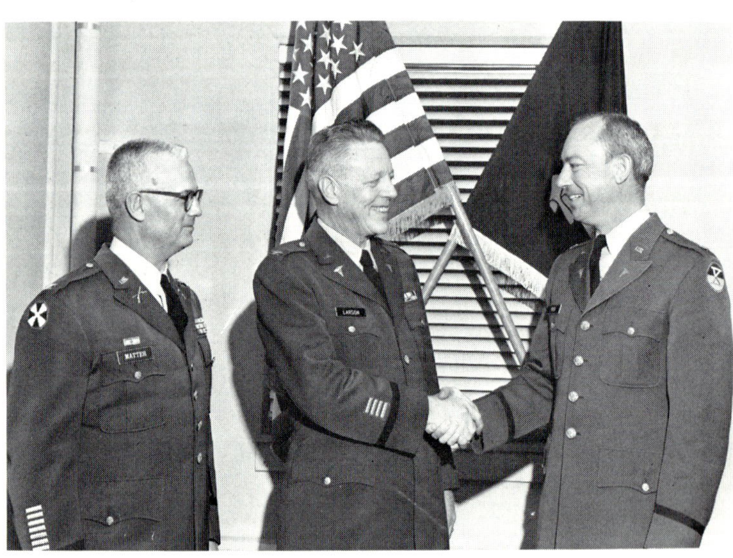

"Crime Doctor" insisted on examining a body at the scene of the crime before any evidence has been disturbed. In 1948 he investigated a rape-murder in the woods near Olympia, Washington.

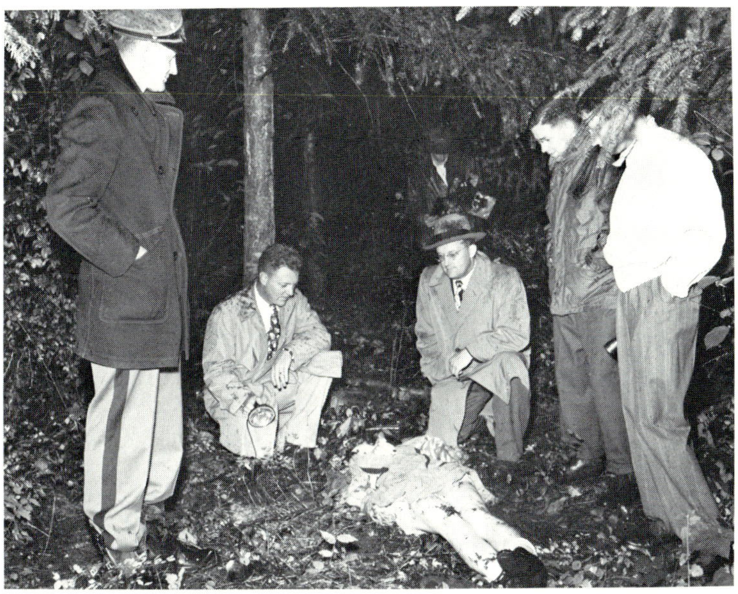

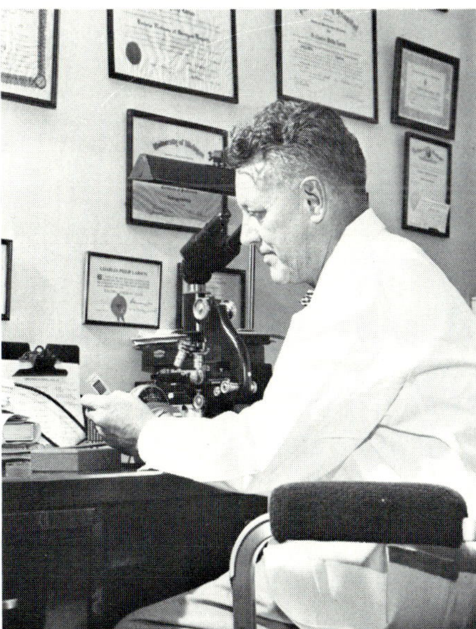

Dr. Larson operated his own independent crime laboratory in the Tacoma General Hospital, Tacoma, Washington. He is now retired.

As president of the National Boxing Association (1961-62), Dr. Larson maintained a continuing interest in boxing that began when he was a student at Gonzaga and was knocked out in his first professional fight. Here he is shown with Floyd Patterson and his manager, Cus D'Amato.

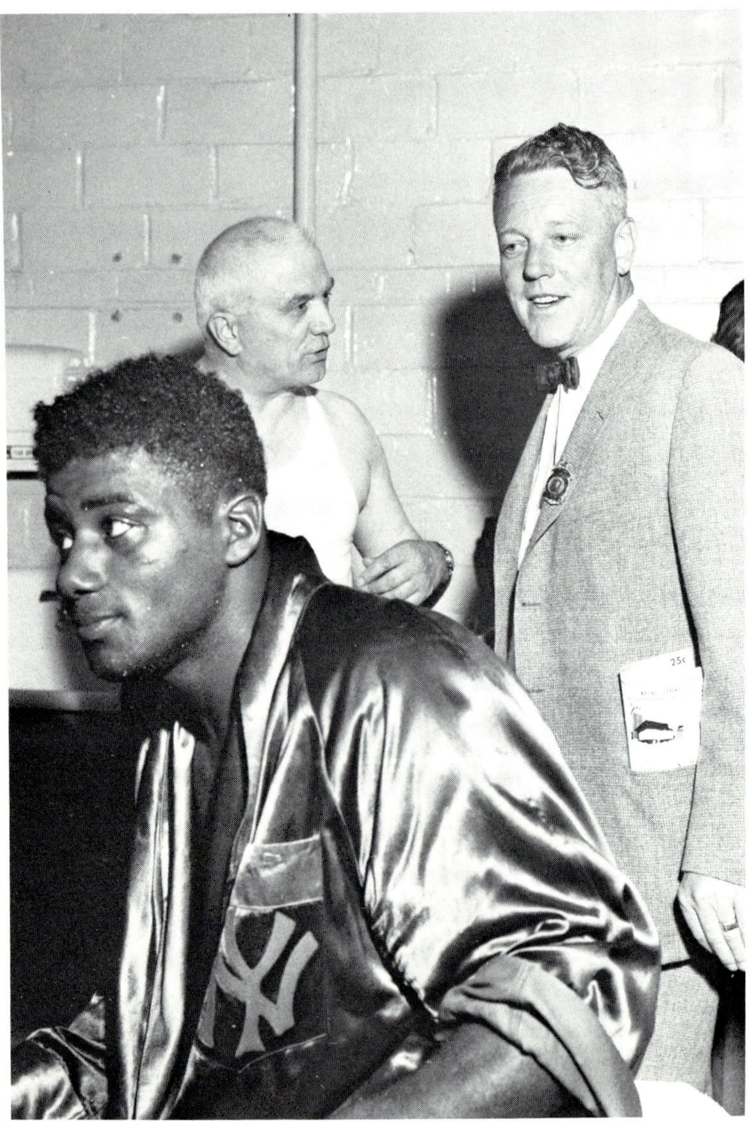

The "Crime Doctor's" laboratory at Tacoma General Hospital was visited in 1958 by Charles Zittel, former Tacoma Chief of Police (center) and Dr. Francis Camps, Chief Pathologist, Scotland Yard, London, England. The exhibits are part of the Tacoma Police Crime Laboratory Museum.

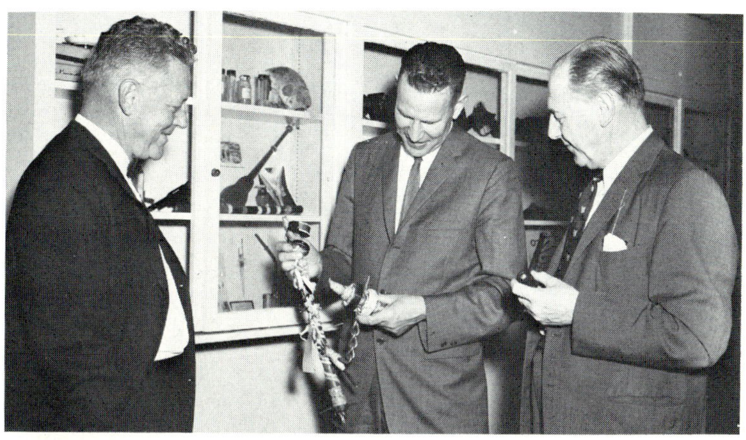

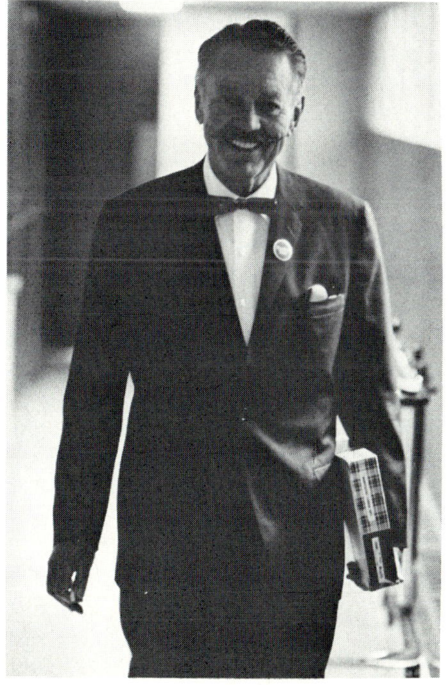

Dr. Larson leaving his office in 1976 sporting his twin trademarks—a neatly shaped handlebar mustache and a thin bow-tie.

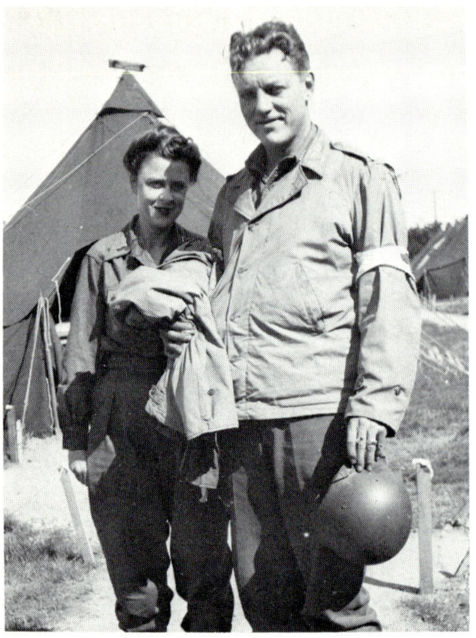

Lt. Margaret Kobervig was a nurse at Camp Carson, Colorado, when she and the then Major Larson first met. After the war they were married, and he established his famous crime lab in Tacoma, Washington.

Family portrait in 1969: Four sons from left to right are Paul, C. Philip, Charles Palmer, and Larry. Seated are three daughters, Elizabeth at the left, Lillian and Christine at the right flanking Margaret and Dr. Charles Larson.

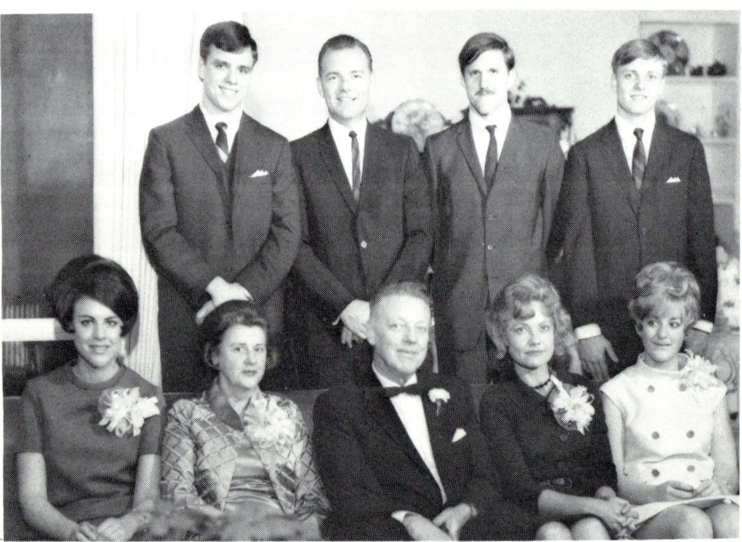

Practically at Tacoma's back door is some of the best salmon fishing in the world. Ken Ollar, a long-time fishing buddy, and Dr. Larson display their catch of salmon at Neah Bay, Washington. Dr. Larson maintains his commercial fishing license.

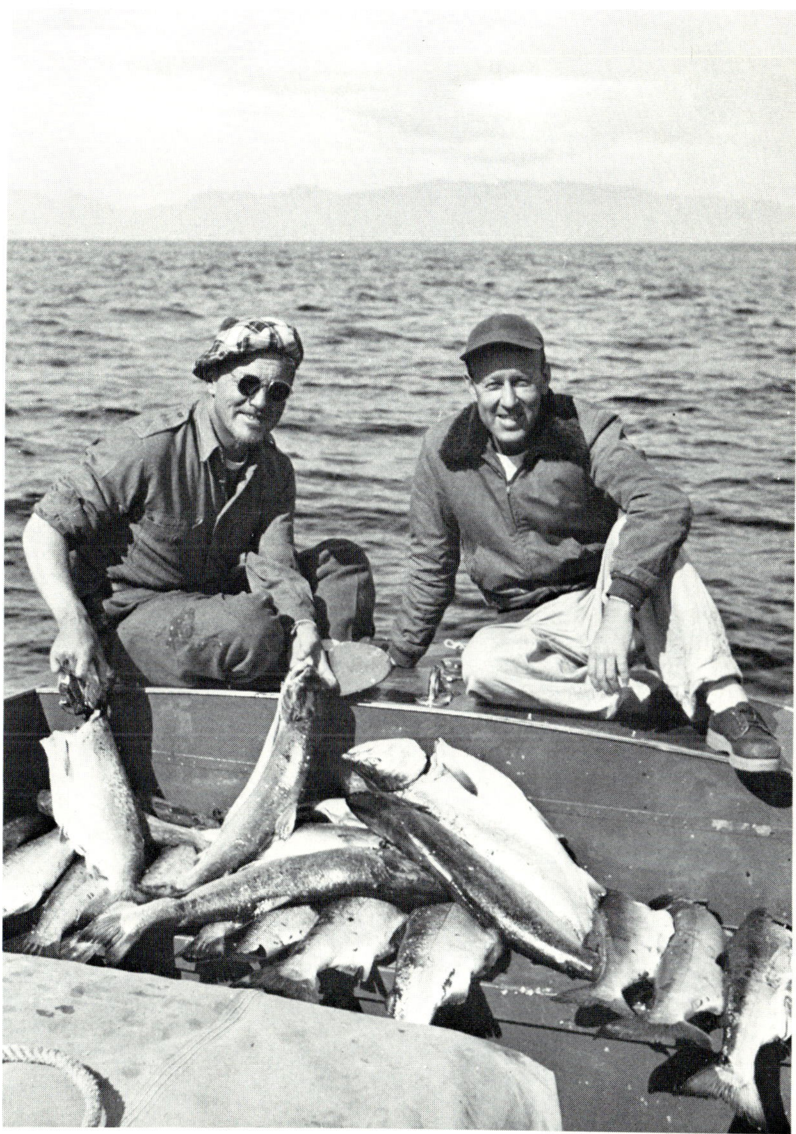

In 1955 Dr. Larson won the fishing derby at the annual convention of the two large national societies of pathology in Miami, Florida. The prize sailfish weighed 92 pounds. His fishing partner is unidentified.

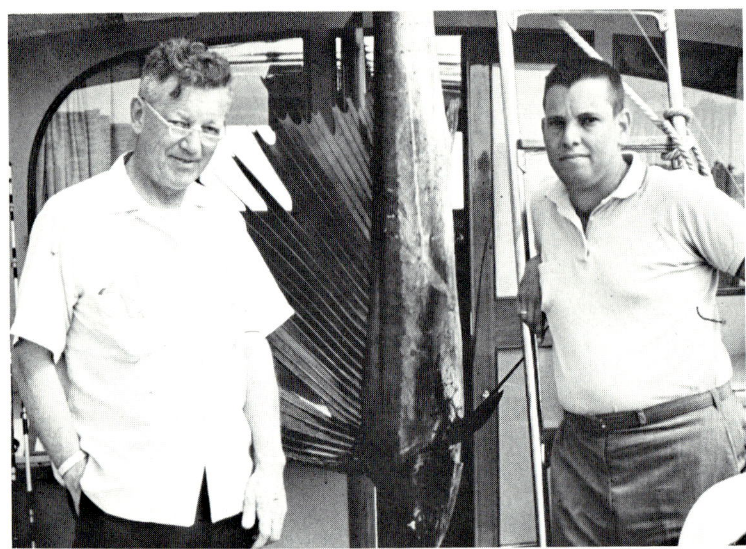

On a fishing trip with his son, C. Philip Larson, Jr., they caught a 48-pound king salmon—plus a few other prizes.

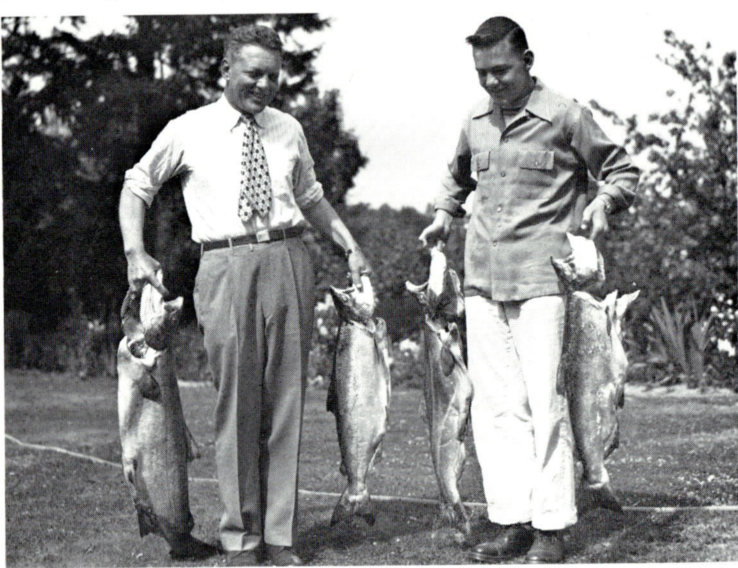

There was indication of the involvement of Jake Bird in murders in Louisville, Kentucky; Omaha, Nebraska; Portage, Wisconsin; Orlando, Florida; Cleveland, Ohio; Evanston, Illinois; Sioux Falls, South Dakota; Kansas City, Kansas—eleven possible killings all around the United States before the murders of the two Kludt women in Tacoma.

At 7 a.m., five hours after the bodies of the two women had been found, Dr. Charles P. Larson had been retained and was at the scene of the crime.

From Larson's notes made at the time:

> The mother had been hit so hard upon the head that the skull had fractured and the dura mater (a sack of membrane which encloses the brain in a cushion of liquid) had been ruptured, so that brain tissue had exuded and was in evidence on the floor and in the matted hair of the victim. The head of a human is like a balloon or a rubber ball filled with putty; you hit it and the putty doesn't compress so it's got to squirt out. Brain tissue is about the consistency of soft putty; if you produce a large depressed fracture in the skull, breaking the membrane or dura mater, then the brain tissue squirts out. I have seen cases in an automobile accident where a man's skull was fractured and brain tissue had squirted 30 feet. I once prepared a demonstration to dramatize this fact to a group of students. I filled a plastic ball with cooked oatmeal, cemented the two halves together to seal the oatmeal in, chilled the ball to make it brittle and then broke into it with the blow of a hammer. After my audience got the oatmeal out of their eyes, ears and hair, they seemed convinced.

Dr. Larson high-tailed it from the murder scene to the County Hospital where Jake Bird was being held in the prison ward and asked for access to his clothing. There were smears on his trouser legs resembling brain tissue and blood on the cuffs that could be human.

At this point in the investigation, Dr. Larson confessed that he was getting as keyed up as a prizefighter before a title match. The Tacoma Police had Jake Bird positioned in the general area in which the Kludt murders had been committed—*but not actually at the scene of the crimes.* He had resisted arrest violently enough to have been beaten into submission by the arresting and custodial officers to a point of hospitalization, a sometimes indication of guilt. Eleven police departments around the country were slowly weaving a web of his implication in 11 other murders. But every bit of it so far was purely circumstantial. None of it was evidence and in the face of that cold fact, there Dr. Larson stood with Jake Bird's filthy pants in his hands.

"It's possible to take material from textiles, make sections of it and see brain cells," Dr. Larson explained. "That doesn't prove that they're human brain cells; you have to do a special test for that, using immune serum. By what's called a precipitin test, you can determine whether your specimens contain human substance or not. If they do, then you can say it's human brain tissue."

Dr. Larson took Jake's pants to his laboratory, made the necessary sections of the stains on the left leg and put them under the microscope.

"Now, brain tissue, under the microscope, has a very characteristic appearance," Dr. Larson said. "No other tissue in the body looks quite like brain tissue. So when you make microscopic sections and study this material, there can be just no question in the mind of a competent man that he's got nerve cells present and that it is brain tissue. It could be brain tissue from an animal, mark you, such as a dog or a cat, but it would be no problem identifying it as brain tissue. But in this case my precipitin test was positive, and this indicated that what I had was human brain tissue, or at least tissue from a primate of the same general species, of which the gorilla is one."

No doubt about it, the stains on the cuffs of Jake Bird's trousers were dried human blood.

Dr. Larson made a Code Three police car run to the morgue and typed the blood from the bodies of Mrs. Kludt and her daughter. Some of the stains on the trouser cuffs were made by the same type of blood as Mrs. Kludt's, and some by the same type as daughter Beverly. In short, before the Kludt murders were 15 hours old, Dr. Larson had enough breaks to pull Jake Bird in out of the cold general area and put him squarely down at the red hot scene of the crimes. There is an exhilaration to the successful working out into incontrovertible fact of a hunch like that. It is comparable to the clout of a double straight bourbon when your ship is safely on the hook and snugly coiled down after a hard day's sail. That—is Dr. Larson's *life.*

The arresting officers had placed Jake Bird in the *area* of the scene of the crime. Dr. Larson had now placed him close enough to the crime—to be *splashed*, by two types of blood, one the type of one dead woman's blood and the second the type of the other's—and by brain tissue.

Dr. Larson readily admitted that there is no known way of identifying the previous owner of brain tissue. Nevertheless, from the head of one of the dead women brain tissue had exuded, and that is as tight an argument as a forensic pathologist can hope to come up with. No one except a pathologist could legitimately have human brain tissue on his pants. "And a sloppy one, at that!" Dr. Larson said.

But it was not tight enough, apparently, for the defense attorney at the subsequent trial. In cross examination he asked Dr. Larson if it was not possible for the brain tissue he had sectioned from Jake Bird's pants to be brain tissue from a gorilla. Apparently the defense attorney had read up on the subject for there is as yet no antiserum that will define human brain tissue from gorilla brain tissue.

Dr. Larson said, "Yes," and gave the defense attorney a long theatrical pause and then said, "But as far as we know, there were no reports of a gorilla running loose in the vicinity of 21st and J Streets at 2:30 in the morning of the night in question—at least, no gorilla who was carrying his shoes in his hand."

Dr. Larson was satisfied that they had their suspect lashed to the mast, especially when his "make" began to connect him with similar crimes around the U.S., but Dr. Larson was short on experience with this sort of criminal, so he made a study in depth of Jake while the opportunity offered.

From his talks with Bird, Dr. Larson concluded that he was a psychopath with a hang-up or fixation on things that caused him sexual excitation and satisfaction. His principal hang-up was that he got a gut-kick from seeing women with expressions of horror and fear on their faces, and he got his orgasms by killing them. Most of them that he did kill were either hatchet or axe murders. They were mostly *white* women, and they were all women he did not know. He hated whites—and he hated women of any color. His thing was to surprise them alone, after watching their homes, or to break in on them in motel rooms. He was a "gandy dancer," a man who works on the railroad, at hard, backslaving work, putting the ties in and repairing and laying new rails.

Jake Bird traveled all around the country continuously. He would come into a city, and two days before the repair train was due to pull out again, he would go around in the neighborhood close to the area where he was working. In the case of the Kludt women it was 20 blocks up the hill from the railroad tracks, and he would peek in the windows. That way he cased the area and set up his marks, usually to be hit his last night in town.

When he entered a house—a house generally with no sign of men around—he usually entered after the woman was in bed. Then very quietly he would take off his shoes and go into the bedroom and axe or bludgeon his victim to death. Never did he attack them sexually. The axe or club was his penis as a hand gun, or a motorcycle is to other mixed-up men.

Afterwards, he would tokenly ransack the house—open the bureau drawers but seldom dump them. He would take money from pocketbooks, put it on a table—and sometimes leave it. A childish effort, one supposes, to make it look as if robbery had been the motive, for sex deviates live in shame and must cover their aberrations. Then, carrying his shoes, he would leave. Mrs. Kludt, however, was conscious enough to scream after he struck her the first time. That scream woke her daughter, so Jake got two victims the last time he prowled.

Basically, Pat Steele, the prosecuting attorney, had a very weak case when he began, and he knew it. All he had was a battered defendant, Bird, and a one-page confession which was recorded a few hours after his arrest.

> My name is Jake Bird. I am 45 years old and was born in Louisiana but haven't had any permanent home since 1920. I quit my job as an extra gang worker on the railroad at Pocatello, Idaho, left there on Wednesday, October 22, and went to Spokane. I came to Seattle from Spokane on Sunday, October 26, 1947, and came to Tacoma on Monday, October 27, 1947. Monday night I got a room at the Elgin Hotel and moved to a different hotel the next day. I didn't use my right name at these hotels, but I don't remember what name I did use.
>
> Sometime the morning in question, after midnight, I left my hotel and went walking, down Broadway, up 17th Street and into the residential district. I was looking for some place that would be easy to go into to burglarize. I was walking up 21st Street and noticed this house at 1007 South 21st and decided to try it. I was going to try the front door but it was too bright, so I decided to try the back door instead. I found the back door unlocked and went inside. Sometime after I went inside, I'm not sure exactly where I put them, but I took off my shoes. I was carrying an axe which I had found in a shed nearby. I carried the axe to bluff anybody off of me that tried to bother me. I set the axe down inside the kitchen near the door. After taking off my shoes so I wouldn't make any noise, I started looking around, and went into a bedroom where a woman was

sleeping. I knew she was sleeping because I could hear her snoring. There was considerable light from the street lights outside, so that I could see my way around, I found a woman's purse on the dresser, picked it up and went out in the kitchen with it to open it. It only had a dollar and a half in it, which I took out and put in my pocket. Correction: I couldn't get the purse opened at first and while I was trying to open it I heard a little noise behind me, looked around and saw a woman standing behind me. I told her that I had a gun and if she started to do anything or holler, I'd shoot. I told her to go on back and get to bed and she wouldn't get hurt. She hesitated and I told her, "You don't have to be afraid of a rape or attack or anything like that, I am only looking for money." Just then the girl came up behind me and grabbed me and I thought it was a boy. The older woman started screaming and grabbed me too, by the arm. I told them to help me find my shoes and I'd leave the house. I broke away and got hold of my axe. They kept on strugglin' with me and the older woman kept screaming, and the girl kept spending her efforts trying to hold me. I finally knocked the big woman down; she didn't fall completely, she started to set down on the floor. The girl let go of me and went over and turned on the light and then she screamed. I was looking around for my shoes. The woman got up off the floor and came back and grabbed me and the girl grabbed me again, too. I just kept on swinging and fighting. After they were down, any blows that I struck was when it appeared to me that they were trying to get up, but I don't remember how many blows I struck, and I don't remember striking any blows after they didn't try to get up any more. I went on looking for my shoes then and went out on the back porch to look for them and went back in again, and finally found them. I took the purse out on the back porch and took the money out of it and was starting to put my shoes on when I saw the police car, or what I thought was a police car, stop and turn off their lights. I grabbed my shoes and ran across the street. They caught me in a yard. I had a knife in my hand and I made a pass at the policeman with it, figuring that he would shoot me and kill me, but he didn't do nothing but call his partner. His partner ran up and I said to him, "Get back, I got a knife," and I figured he'd shoot, too, but he didn't. They finally got me down on the ground, and arrested me.

I was beaten up by the police officers, about the head and face, mouth, side, before I was taken to the hospital.

I make this statement because I want Mr. Mann and Mr. Lyons to have all the facts and the truth. I have not been mistreated by them and no promises nor duress have been used to get me to make this statement. I know that this statement can be used against me.

Signed: Jake Bird

Actually, Bird's confession did not tell Steele a whole lot, though it was of some help. He also had psychiatrist Dr. George Rickle's opinion that Jake was of sound mind when he signed the statement. But there was nothing to corroborate the Kludt killings. Steele had all the evidence, but he had no fingerprints. He had Bird's trousers, jacket, a pair of shoes—he had a patent leather purse from the death scene with no fingerprints. He told Dr. Larson, "This case is in terrible shape. I wish there was something I could hang my hat on—a fingerprint or a blood type or something."

By now Dr. Larson was on the case, and six days after Bird had been captured, Steele received a call from Larson.

"Well, you can quit worrying," Dr. Larson said.

"What did you find?" Steele asked.

"Brain tissue," Dr. Larson said. "I found human brain tissue on Bird's pants, jacket, shoes and the axe."

While it was a big breakthrough, Steele still had problems. When he was lining up the police officers to testify at the trial, he discovered that nobody had marked any of the evidence. None of the pieces had been properly identified. There wasn't any question that the articles were the same, but the officers had not chalked them so that they could honestly look at them and say, "Yes, this is my mark; yes, this is the object that I handled."

Steele asked Officer Skip Davies, "How'd you mark the shoes?" And Davies replied, "I never marked the shoes." And Steele told him, "Now, listen, Skip, when I hand you those shoes, you'd better find something that tells you these are the shoes you found on the fence across the street from the Kludt home. Right?" "Right."

Patrolman Sabutis had handled the trousers and shirt. Steele asked him, "Did you mark them, Tiny?" Sabutis said, "No, I'll go put my mark on them right now." And Steele said, "Don't you dare touch them."

That was the sort of nonsense Prosecuting Attorney Pat Steele had to contend with.

The Trial

THE doctor was precise and confident. He clipped the tips from four stems of asparagus with one stroke of the knife. He chewed in careful cadence and his conversation was as sharply defined as his shoulders, which are square and still muscular.

"To win Jake's confidence," Dr. Larson said, addressing himself more to my tape cassette than to me, "an attorney had to be able to defend himself."

"Why?" I said. It is a reporter's best word.

"Jake knew a lot of law."

"Where did he learn law?"

"He didn't learn law. He *read* about the law. In prison libraries. He had spent 12 years in a Utah prison. Twelve years in a penitentiary in Iowa. Five more years in the pen at Jackson, Michigan. Mentally, he was sharp as a tack, an avid reader, an able conversationalist and witty. I tell you, he was a very *sophisticated* burglar. He could talk you right out of your socks."

"Talkative, then?"

"Oh, yes. He loved to talk. He'd tell you anything you wanted to hear—and more. He was very calculating."

"Was Jake capable of being remorseful?"

"I don't think so. Killing was second nature to him. He snuffed out human life the way you'd mash a fly. It didn't seem to bother him at all. He hated white people. As a young man, he'd been thwarted in some long-ago love affair with a white girl back in his home town of Greenwood, Louisiana. Rather than find himself hanging from a limb of a tree, he joined a carnival as a handyman and hit the road. After that and for the rest of his life, he lived the life of a man constantly on the move. Along the way he managed to stuff enough formal education into himself to amount to what was comparable to a high school education. But I can tell you this, Jake Bird was an *educated* man. He got a lot of it all up and down the line, particularly in prison libraries."

"He seemed to be a man of many personalities."

"You never could tell about him. Pat Steele told me about talking to a district attorney in Lincoln County in Nebraska about Jake. The DA's name was Hollister. Jake had been a witness for him in a murder trial against a brakeman of the Burlington Railroad who had, according to Jake, struck and killed this 18-year-old boy on a freight train. The boy happened to be the son of a very wealthy Cleveland publishing family—some branch of the Hearst family. So Jake was the prime witness, and he was given the red-carpet treatment while awaiting trial. Later, when Pat wrote to Hollister asking for his recollections of Jake, he wrote back saying what a mannerly, courteous fellow Jake had been. Why, he'd even had Jake out to his home for dinner a couple of times while preparing his case. He was very impressed with Jake."

"Were you?"

"Oh, yes. Jake was a very fascinating fellow. Dangerous as sin, but fascinating."

At lunch the next day, I trimmed the broiled fat from around my steak. I have always been a patient man; I had spent 30 of my 53 years trying to locate facts and then to reduce them to words. I wanted a lot of facts from Pat Steele.

"Are you the one who dubbed Dr. Larson the Crime Doctor?"

The former District Attorney of Pierce County sipped coffee and nodded.

"Yes," Steele said. "I started calling him that during the Bird trial."

"When did you first meet him?"

"In the fall of '47, maybe sooner. Anytime there was a murder we called Dr. Larson. I don't care who you're talking about, he's one of the most preeminent forensic pathologists in the world."

"A damned good man to have on your side."

Pat Steele looked up and smiled.

"A perfect witness," he said. "All his career he has been retained at fairly stiff fees not only to present the truth but to convince juries that what he tells them *is* the truth."

"His testimony made the difference in the Bird trial."

"He never once looked at Jake while he was on the stand," Steele remembered. "He focused all his attention on the jury. He has a system of testifying that he has used for 30 years. He has the conviction that if a scientist is going to testify to a jury, and he knows his testimony is purely objective, true and correct, he has an obligation to *educate* the jury and to tell the jury, in terms they can understand, the true facts about the case. Therefore, if he has something to tell the jury, he approaches them in somewhat the way a salesman does, opening slowly with the soft sell first. He feels he has a definite obligation to portray to the jury exactly what he has done in his investigation, what scientific methods he has used to arrive at his conclusions, to convince them that he is correct in those conclusions."

Because I had talked to Dr. Larson about his courtroom style only 24 hours earlier, I said, "When he faces a jury for the first time, he says he makes it a practice to take a good, long look at the 12 members and size them up during the time that his qualifications are being reviewed."

"He gets on that stand and you course him along through the proceedings—and he looks at that jury—he ponders your question momentarily—and then he lays it out," Steele said. "He talks to each juror in turn—he goes up and down the jury box like he's playing a pipe organ. It takes about a half-hour to establish the qualifications of an expert witness, and during that time Dr. Larson answers a lot of questions about where he went to medical school, where he trained, etcetera. During that half-hour he scans the jury, sizing them up, to see who's really going to be interested in what he has to say—and who is just bored. At the same time he is forming in his own mind an opinion about each juror. So before he is finished being qualified, he has had a chance to study all 'tried-and-true' 12 of them. When he begins his testimony then, he talks to one juror at a time, riveting his eyes on his or hers until he is sure he has him interested and then he moves his attention to another juror. He skips his attention around, he doesn't go right down the line, because he doesn't want what he is doing to be obvious. He talks directly to one juror at a time, putting his testimony on a person-to-person basis, until he is sure in his own mind that each one is thoroughly convinced. Whether this method hurts—or helps—the defendant is not his concern. His only obligation is to be sure that the jury clearly understands what has been done, and what is fact and what is not fact. He testifies only in fields in which he is an expert."

"Dr. Larson said that when he was very young and starting out," I said, "he ranged out of his field several times and got crucified. He said you can't do this, because when you're proven wrong, your impact upon the jury is completely lost. They lose all confidence in you."

"In the Bird trial," Steele said, "Dr. Larson told the jury how both women died. He explained that Bertha

Kludt died not from the head injuries but from the fact that her windpipe had been slashed completely across with a dull instrument, apparently an axe. She'd been hit on the head several times and was lying down when the axe was used to sever her windpipe. The murder weapon, the axe, was a prosecution exhibit in the jury room."

"Even though he signed a confession," I said, "Bird changed his story and claimed he didn't kill the Kludt women. You talked to him numerous times, what did he say to you?"

"This was the version he gave me," Steele said. "He went to the house to rob it. This was not a sex murder, let me make that clear. It was strictly a case of burglary. He was a *house* burglar, not a store burglar. That was his specialty—houses. His style was to prowl the neighborhoods, find an open door and walk in armed with a piece of pipe, knife or an axe to protect himself. It was something of a ritual. He'd go into a house, he'd listen for any movement, take a measurement of the area, turn on a light and look around. Then he'd take off his shoes and set them against the back door, with his axe leaning against the back wall of the kitchen.

"At the Kludt home he saw Mrs. Kludt's bedroom off to the left of the kitchen. She was asleep and he could see her handbag. He crept in, took the handbag, and then went back to the kitchen and emptied the contents on the table. He was standing there sorting out the stuff when Mrs. Kludt awoke, got up, saw Jake in the kitchen, and rushed him. In his version of what happened next, he said he was struggling with the mother when the daughter Beverly suddenly appeared. She had been asleep upstairs, heard the commotion, slipped down the stairs and into the kitchen, and jumped Jake from behind. Jake later admitted to me that between the two of them they almost overpowered him. He said he had an awful time getting to his axe. But he managed to get to it, flailed it around and finally subdued the women. In the melee he crushed Beverly's skull, with brain tissue flying out of the fracture and splashing on his pants. Then he turned on Mrs. Kludt and finished her off."

It was impossible, Steele said, for Bird to explain logically how he got human brain tissue on his pants. He neither denied nor admitted he was even at the scene of the murders, and later rejected the argument that he had signed the confession voluntarily. He claimed he was *forced* to sign it without the benefit of a lawyer.

"But tell me," Steele pointed out, "how could an itinerant worker, a black man—how could he possibly explain the human brain tissue on his pants? He couldn't even explain the presence of brain tissue, let alone *human* brain tissue."

Charles Zittle, then a detective lieutenant, remembers Jake's trial. He particularly remembers when John Hickey was put on the stand to testify. Hickey was the police officer who had beaten Bird to a pulp in the police paddy-wagon.

"Jake's appearance was a fright," Zittle recalls. "There was no denying that Hickey had worked him over. After he'd seen what Jake had done to the two women, John just seemed to go berserk. At the trial Pat Steele decided to admit the beating. Jim Selden, one of the two defense attorneys, tried to make an issue out of it. At one point in Hickey's testimony, he told Selden he didn't consider Jake a man. Selden jumped on that fast. 'Well,' he said, 'what *do* you consider him?' And Hickey said, 'A beast.' Selden dropped that line of questioning right now.

"Thank god," Zittle said, "for Dr. Larson. If it hadn't been for his testimony, Jake Bird would have been back on the street killing people again."

In his testimony, Dr. Larson felt it was an open-and-shut case and told the jury so. The evidence against Jake was so compelling that they couldn't do anything else but find him guilty, the doctor said. When he finished testifying, there was no cross-examination. Judge Ed Hodge took a recess and asked Steele and the two defense attorneys to join him in his chambers. Closing the door after them, the judge chuckled. "Well, Jim," he said to Jim Selden, "I thought you'd probably want another hour of cross-examination." Selden frowned. "I wouldn't walk into that trap, Judge," he said.

Dr. Larson had nailed the defense to the cross.

He had left the defense with very little argument.

He had all but wrapped Jake Bird in a coffin.

Without putting Jake on the stand, the only recourse the defense had was to highlight a review of the testimony. In retrospect, Pat Steele feels that it was a mistake for Bird not to have taken the stand in his own defense.

"Had he taken the stand he might have left a question of doubt in somebody's mind on that jury," Steele said. "He was a most persuasive, most articulate actor. Several days before he came to trial, he told Sig Kittleson, chief criminal deputy, that he wanted to talk to me. It was urgent, he said. I went right down to the jail house to find out what was on his mind. He began the conversation with a long, drawn-out tale about wanting to live. 'Mr. Steele,' he said, 'I don't want to die. I don't want to hang. I want to live.' He was bargaining now for his life. He was *always* bargaining, sparring for time. He had it figured out that possibly I would buy his plea of guilty to two first-degree murders in exchange for consecutive life sentences. I told him, 'I can't do anything like that.' Unfortunately, the word got out that Jake was bartering for his life. The rumor led to big headlines: 'BIRD MAY GET OFF WITH LIFE.' I squelched that story fast."

The jury of nine men and three women took only 35 minutes to come to a verdict. Bird was found guilty of two counts of first-degree murder.

Eleven days later, on December 6, 1947, only 37 days after killing the Kludts, he was back in Judge E. D. Hodge's court for sentencing. This time the room was virtually empty. Only those who had participated in the trial were present—plus Bill Dugovich, the only news reporter there.

Selden and Paulsen, Bird's attorneys, must have known all the way what the verdict would be. Selden, with cool detachment, told the judge in his final argument that there was nothing more he could add in his client's defense. Paulsen was more dramatic. Bound by legal ethics, he made a final argument for Bird's life.

Judge Hodge listened quietly, and when Paulsen had finished, he turned to Bird, who was wearing an old woolen shirt and faded khaki trousers, and said, "Mr. Bird, is there anything you have to say before sentencing."

From behind the defendant's table, Jake pulled himself erect. "Your Honor," he said. "I did not commit any crime. I am not guilty. I killed nobody. I signed that confession you have only to save my own life. The *police* made me do it."

This was the first time Jake had addressed the court. During the trial his defense attorneys refused to let him take the stand. But Jake wasn't through having his say:

"Your Honor," he continued, pointing to his tattered prison garments, "just look how nicely clothed I am. Just notice how well I've been taken care of." He seethed with sarcasm. "Look at the teeth I don't have anymore." He opened his mouth and revealed one mangled fang above and below. He fingered the hole in his nose where the police had punched it out with their Billy clubs. "Yes, sir," he told Judge Hodge, "I sure been treated wonderful by the City of Tacoma—"

Suddenly there was a scream at the back of the courtroom. A woman jumped to her feet and shouted, "Let that man go! He is not guilty! He is innocent!" An embarrassed hush fell over the room. The woman was quickly escorted out. Jake continued.

Now he dropped his bomb. "All of you," he said, gazing from face to face, " who have had anything to do with my case will be punished. I am putting the Jake Bird hex on you. Mark my words, you will die before I do."

The judge slammed his gavel on the bar.

"That'll be enough, Mr. Bird. You've had your say. Now I will have mine."

Here it came.

"On January 16th, 1948, at precisely one minute past midnight, I sentence you to be hung by the neck until dead. The sentence will be carried out at the Washington State Penitentiary, Walla Walla."

The State wasn't wasting any time.

When the death penalty was read, Jake's only emotion was to blink. He was perfectly silent. Five deputy sheriffs surrounded him and ushered him out of the courtroom and back to his cell down the street. While he said nothing, you knew his head was spinning.

On January 2nd Bill Dugovich was in the office of Undersheriff Joe Karpach trying to pry new information out of him concerning Bird. Karpach made the claim that Jake had just confessed to several more murders. "About six or seven more," Karpach said. Bill sensed the story was growing bigger all the time. The real viciousness of the condemned man was unfolding daily.

The next day, a Saturday, Karpach admitted to Bill that the number of confessed murders by Bird had risen to 10 over 20 years. Again, the *Tacoma News Tribune* had a page one headline story.

Late that afternoon, Dugovich went to his managing editor, J. Ernest Knight, and asked permission to call Olympia to talk to Governor Mon C. Wallgren about a possible reprieve for Bird.

"I don't think you'll find the governor in," Ernie Knight said, "but go ahead and try."

Governor Wallgren answered immediately. Bill put the question to him.

"A stay of execution may be granted to clean up other murders," Governor Wallgren said. "However, if we see that the confessions are lies, we will not grant any delays."

Dugovich tried to talk to Bird several times, but the sheriff wouldn't allow him near Jake. "He's too dangerous, Bill," the sheriff said.

"So I never talked to him," Dugovich said. "Later, others got to him—reporters Jim Faber and Jack Pyle and, of course, Frank Herbert—but I missed. At first, we were told by police that Jake was dumb, illiterate and that he lied a lot. So they didn't want the press near him. Actually, Jake proved to be an eloquent speaker, a voracious reader of law books and the possessor of a phenomenal memory."

The Jake Bird hex? Was it a hoax? You figure it out. Judge Hodge, who'd been in excellent health, died one month after sentencing Jake. Before January ran itself out, Joe Karpach dropped dead of a heart attack. Chief Court Clerk Ray Scott was buried in February—also of heart failure. Six months afterward Police Lt. Sherman Lyons, who had obtained Bird's confession, died—again of a coronary. The next one to go was one of Jake's attorneys, J. W. Selden. He died on the anniversary of Jake's sentencing. Assigned to defend Jake against his own wishes, Selden had told the jury during the trial: "My heart does not beat in sympathy for this man, who fixed his life as more important than that of others." The sixth man to die by Bird's so-called "hex" was Arthur A. Stoward. Arthur had been one of Jake's guards at Walla Walla.

The only two that Jake's hex didn't affect were Pat Steele and Dr. Larson.

"Jake didn't put his so-called hex on me personally," Dr. Larson remembers. "The way I found out about it was from Pat Steele. Pat walked into my lab one day and said that he and I, among others, were hexed; that Jake had predicted we were going to die within the year. We both laughed and went out and had a drink on it. The fact that Pat and I were the only two out of eight who survived is a matter of pure coincidence. Those six men who did die didn't die of Jake Bird, they died of coronary occlusions."

In his practice throughout the years, Dr. Larson has helped convict in courts of homicide, he estimates, about 100 men. A number of these men have threatened to kill him in reprisal. It never occurred to him to remember their names or when they *would* get out, or to take any precautionary measures if he happened to be told when they did get out. "The desire for revenge is a very immature reaction," he says, "and whereas your average murderer is seldom a very mature, well-rounded character, he is nevertheless subject to the cooling process—the changes that come with the passage of time. Come to think of it, that's what our penal system is all about, isn't it—to put people on the shelf until they cool off?"

Dr. Larson chuckled softly. "I like the thought, anyway."

Sing Like a Bird

IT took me a little while," Dr. Larson said, "to see Jake Bird as a complex person." He reached for the sugar for his coffee. "Now there was a bright boy," he said earnestly. "I mean really bright. And yet, he chose a life that cost him more than half his life in jail."

"And finally his life," I said. "How many people did Jake actually kill?"

"The estimates went as high as 44," Dr. Larson said. "He got what he deserved."

The death sentence was read in Tacoma on December 6, 1948. The following day he was whisked away to the state penitentiary at Walla Walla, where he was scheduled to die at midnight, January 16.

"On the way to prison," the doctor said, "Jake strung out Joe Karpach, from the Pierce County sheriff's office, about all those unsolved murder cases he could clear up. Joe, of course, envisioned himself in the role of hero; he didn't realize that Jake was just sparring for time. Sure, there was a lot Jake could talk about that was authentic—a lot he could talk about that could excite your interest if he thought it would buy him time. So he'd spin off a lot of stories."

"Who was the warden at Walla Walla at the time?"

"Tom Smith. He told Pat Steele that Jake came into the prison talking a blue streak. The first thing he wanted was pencil and paper and stamp, and he wrote back to Judge Hodge: 'I appeal my conviction,' and he signed it Jake Bird. *That* was his appeal. However, Judge Hodge ruled that the clerk didn't have to accept Jake's notice of appeal."

In the shadow of the noose Bird took a long look at the calendar, and with but a few weeks before he was to die, he sent word to Warden Smith that he wanted to talk "to clear my conscience." He said he could solve for authorities at least ten murders, maybe more. Warden Smith phoned Pat Steele and Detective Lieutenant Sherman Lyons of the Tacoma Police Department and invited them to come over and listen.

Before leaving Tacoma, Steele told the press: "I want to give Jake a chance to tell what he knows, but I don't intend to permit him to use what he might have withheld as a means to add a few days to his life. I won't ask for a stay of execution unless it seems absolutely necessary."

Pat Steele, accompanied by Lt. Lyons and a court reporter, sat across a table from Bird at the state prison and looked him straight in the eyes.

"Okay, Jake," he said, "where do you want to start?"

"Well," Jake said, "I told the warden this morning that I have never backed down on a deal in my life, and I do not intend to back down on this one. I told him that if he appointed me a lawyer to try to appeal my case and get me a stay of execution, I will tell all. The warden told me to proceed with cases I though should be cleared up."

"Where do you want to start, Jake?" Steele repeated.

"Well," Jake replied, "let's begin with a fellow named Clarence Lukehart. He was convicted for murder in 1928.

Actually, it wasn't a murder at all, even though he pleaded guilty; it was an accidental death, caused by me. It was on a Sunday morning about 10 a.m. I was crossing the railroad tracks near a little place called East Omaha, Iowa, when this kid, about seven or eight, came up behind me and started shouting, 'nigger, nigger, nigger!' I picked up this rock and threw it at him. I did not realize I hit him until I heard him groaning. I went back and picked him up and carried him about 20 feet off the road. Well, there was a clump of bushes growing there, but they wasn't tall enough to hide behind; anybody passing by could see me standing up, so I had to lay down with the kid, who remained unconscious. I tried all day to revive him. At night it rained, and I went and got a blanket and covered him up. The next morning, he was dead."

"What did you do with the body?" Steele asked.

"I had stolen a gun several days before," Jake said, "and when I realized he was dead, I took off all his clothes, hid 'em in this old can I found, and then I hit him over the head a couple of times with the gun. I did that in order to make people think that some kind of fiend did it."

"Where'd you put the body?" Steele asked.

"I just left it there."

"Where did you go?"

"I joined a carnival that was in town and went to Denver. I returned to East Omaha in two weeks and saw in the paper where this convict had confessed to killing the kid. I simply couldn't believe it. He was brought back from Anamosa Reformatory to stand trial. I went to the hearing and I think I would have confessed if the man had gotten the death penalty; that is what he demanded, but the Judge refused and, naturally, I felt better. I tried to figure out some way to say I done it without being caught, but I couldn't figure nothing. Soon after that I got in trouble again and was sent to Ford Madison."

"Let me review your story," Steele said. "You said that

you returned to where the boy was in the evening on account of the rain, and you brought a blanket to cover him. Where did you get the blanket, Jake?"

"I didn't say that," Jake said.

"Well, maybe I misunderstood," Steele said. "What did you say?"

"I said it rained that night and I went and got a blanket."

"Where did you get the blanket?"

"I got it out of my room. No, I got it out of a boxcar. I took all my belongings the morning I met this boy, because I was going to join the carnival, and I had all my belongings, including this blanket and two suitcases, and I had left them in a boxcar over there where they don't use the Union Pacific."

"Now, you said that you returned the next day with this stolen gun and hit the boy in the head several times with it."

"That is right."

"What color hair did the boy have?"

Jake shook his head.

"I don't know," he said.

"You don't know?" Steele said.

"Would you pay any attention to anybody's hair?" Jake said. "I didn't know what color yours was until you mentioned it."

"If I hit somebody in the head, I would know what color the hair was," Steele said. "You returned the next day, broad daylight and hit him several times."

"Oh, you are just assuming things now," Jake said. "You can't tell me that if you hit a man in the head you would know what color his hair was, because you would not be interested in a man's hair. I was out there all night trying to bring the kid to, trying to keep him from dying. I just couldn't believe he was dead. I wouldn't be looking at the color of his hair."

"Okay," Steele said. "Now, you said you attended the trial of Lukehart, is that right?"

"I didn't go inside," hedged Jake. "I was over around the courtroom, yes."

"You didn't go in, you didn't listen to any of the testimony?"

"No."

"You don't know who testified?"

"Well," Jake said, "I think that the warden of the penitentiary and some reporters testified, if I make no mistake."

"Did the boy's mother testify?"

"I did not hear anybody testify. I told you I merely went over around the courthouse to see what the outcome of the judge's sentence was going to be."

"You say that you carried the boy about 20 or 30 feet back into some bushes. Well, when you carried him that distance, was there anybody or anything coming down the road?"

"There was several cars going back and forth," Jake recalled. "And there was a man and a woman coming, walking down the road. I didn't want to be found with the gun on me so I threw it into this low, weedy, watery swamp. It is down there yet, I guess. Then I stopped and looked back to see what this man and woman would do, because the boy was groaning. When they got close to where the boy was laying, they both paused and apparently was trying to find where the noise was coming from, but they finally walked on."

After another hour of routine questioning about the boy's death, Pat Steele called for a recess to lunch. At 2 p.m. the interview was resumed. Jake was still in good form.

"You see, naturally I understand the position you're in," Jake said. "I know none of this in the record is personal, because I don't think you care that much about something that happened 20 years ago. People are saying I am not doing a damn thing now but trying to stall for time, which is true in a way. I am not stalling for time, but still I want time. Regardless of what I say about another case and another state, it has no bearing on what I am convicted on here. A lot of people don't realize that, it seems. But I got letters from lawyers that I would like to hear from further before I die, and I got some things I want to say, because I don't think I got a fair deal."

"Is there anything else you want to tell us about the boy's death?" Steele asked, anxious to move on.

"If you are going to check on what I told you, if you think that is worth me putting down and signing a sworn statement to it, I will do it," Jake said.

"I asked you this morning if you would swear to this statement, and you said no," Steele reminded him. "We are now having it typed up as fast as we can type it, and we will appreciate your signing it if you want to. We can't force you to sign it. But in view of my instructions from the governor, I advise you to tell us fully and completely everything you have to say about it, make it a sworn statement and sign it so that if it is going to get action from the governor, it will just be that much quicker to accomplish the action, either for a stay or reprieve or commutation, whatever it is."

Steele knew of at least eight other crimes involving Jake, and he wanted him to talk about those.

"It is easy for you to pry questions," Jake said.

"I am not trying to pry you, Jake," Steele said. "I am merely giving you an opportunity to relate in toto."

"Well," Jake said, "there is one thing I want to say. If you had not got in such a big hurry to get me hung and over with—well, you will just have to go and do it. You must remember I am not represented at all in none of this. You all have thousands of millions of dollars to back you up; I have not even got a lawyer or nothing. I just got to say what I think is best for me, and I have told you that I committed ten crimes and could prove every one of them, and that is exactly what I will do if given time."

"Well," Steele said, "we would like to clean up those cases so you can get your conscience clear."

"My conscience don't hurt me. I wish you would quit putting in the papers that my conscience is hurting me, because I ain't got no conscience."

"I didn't put it in," Steele said. "I've been too busy with other burglaries to even talk to the papers."

At that point, all but Steele got up and left the room, leaving him alone with Jake.

Jake looked into Steele's face.

"I want you to give a report to the governor." he said.

"This is my report, Jake," Steele said, fingering a large folder of papers. "It comes from my court reporter, who has been taking everything down. I am not trusting my memory about a thing."

"The thing I want you to tell the Washington governor," Jake said, "is that regardless of what has been said about other crimes in other states, I am just not free to talk now as I want to. As slim a chance as I've got for commuting my sentence, I have got to ask the governor to do it, and I want to tell him further that there has never been a man in the history of Washington who has been given the runaround without benefit of counsel, without a chance of having his day in court and I am asking for my case to be appealed, and counting on lawyers to represent me; one that would at least plead for my life and not get up and tell them to bring in a count of guilty, and tell the judge I should tell the governor—that as bad as my case is in Tacoma, that nobody ever mentioned the statement that I said I would go to the gallows for it, and tell him that I still feel I should have counsel in this case. Tell him about the stay of execution that I am trying to get, about a representative of the law who will represent me. Tell him I appreciate anything he can do for me, that I should have a day in court, and I got to presume that is asking for mercy. I want to tell him also that when Selden argued for a new motion, argued for a new—"

"Motion for a new trial," Steel interposed.

"Yes," Jake said, "arguing for a motion for a new trial, told the jury that I should hang and showed no sympathy for me. Tell the governor I don't think that is hardly the way to argue a motion for a new trial. Tell him when they sentenced me, before I could get my equilibrium and balance and ask the court to appoint me another lawyer, that they rushed me right over here to Walla Walla. Tell him that on the 9th of December I wrote the trial judge and asked for counsel. Tell him the answer was, 'I don't feel at this time that I could grant your request.' Tell him that on the 9th of December I wrote a written motion up there, notice of appeal, a written notice of appeal. Tell him I got no answer from them. Tell him that on the 19th I wrote another letter to the clerk of the court. Tell him that on the 29th of December I got a letter from the clerk telling me if I signed a pauper's oath I could get the necessary records of my trial in order to go ahead. But tell the governor that although I signed the pauper's oath on December 30th and sent them to the court, I still do not have the records in my hand on this, January 6th. Then, I want you to tell him whether, in your opinion, you think that is fair or not.

"You say you are here to represent the governor and see that fair play takes place. I am not going to tell you what to tell him. In your own words tell it to him. Tell him that I also think whether the court is forced to appoint a lawyer for an appeal or not, that I think any place where the death penalty is inflicted, and where there might be errors in the record, and where a man's counsel quit him at the bar, that the State should be ashamed to talk about what little money it would take to hire a lawyer for him to appeal. And tell him that this execution be stayed to investigate further these murders, that he grant this execution stay, that some of it ought to be take up to see whether or not I got a square deal in this matter.

"I want you to further tell the governor that I have not claimed an accomplice in no case where I did not have an accomplice. Tell him that nobody in Tacoma and in the State of Washington will listen to me when I say I had an accomplice in the Tacoma case, because they are not interested in it. They are convinced that I am the murderer. Tell him that is a lie. I feel if I could get my case appealed or a new trial, or some lawyers to argue my case, that I may get clemency. But tell him that if he is only interested in me hanging because the public is clamoring for it and not interested in clearing up all these other cases, then after I am dead I certainly cannot clear them up."

"For the record, Jake," broke in Steele, "those communications you mentioned having sent up there, I received none. I received no communications or any copies. Did you send anything to me or to my office?"

"I did not," said Jake.

"There is another point in there," Steele continued. "You say that at the time you were talking, or something up there, you would go to the gallows with a statement of a certain kind."

"That's correct," said Jake.

"Well," Steele said, "what was that statement? I don't recall you mentioning it."

"Well, I went out the night before the Tacoma killings with a boy from Seattle," Jake explained. "I paid his fare to Tacoma. We went out that night to burglarize some places. The next night we went out again, and I took one side of the street and he took the other. He met me at the Kludt home. When I heard screaming in the house I ran into the house and stumbled over this girl's body in the dining room, and I asked my buddy what took place. He said, 'Hell's broke loose!' But as I was coming up to the back door, he was rushing out of the house and throwed the pocketbook and an axe, and then went back in the house. When I got in the house he was in the parlor, and I said, 'What is going on here?' That's when he said, 'Hell's broken loose!' And I said, 'Hell certainly has broke loose. I'm gettin' the hell outta here!' I went outside, put on my shoes, just as the police car drove up and stopped down the street. I seen two flashlights sweeping around, and my friend took off. I hollered at him but he ran. I believe that's why the police did not grab him, because I hollered. They ran right by him. And that's the truth. I don't care what was on my pants. I don't care if the officers said they saw me running out of the house. The only thing that matters is the *truth.*"

"Did you go out the front or back door, Jake?" Steele asked.

"I ran out the back door when a woman first screamed," Jake said. "I thought it was on the same street that I was on, so a light went on down the street in the upper story. I tried to see around there. I said, 'Well, I can't see a thing, no way.' I looked up at this little house, the lights was on in the back of it, and I started to approach it cautiously, but when I got about 30 feet from the back door, my friend hurried out the back door with the purse and axe in his hand and throwed 'em outside. Now, I don't care whether you believe me or not, but that is the truth. It would be senseless for me to try to involve anybody that is not involved."

At that moment, Warden Smith walked in and joined the discussion. It was plain he had little sympathy for Jake. His patience was running dry.

"Take a look at it this way," he told Jake. "I mean, here are these crimes that have happened over the last 20 years. You say men have gone to prison for offenses you've committed. Some of these cases we want to know about have not been solved after all these years, but if we are going to be sparring around trading back and forth from now on, why it is not going to make too much difference to our governor, to Mr. Steele, or to me whether they are ever solved or not. We just can't drag this thing out forever. I will be honest with you in saying that I don't think that you can possibly get any commutation unless you can make some showing, give us something concrete to work on, involving these other cases. It's your only hope, Jake."

"Come on, Jake, let's get to some of these other things," Steele added. "Let's have the date, the city and the disastrous things."

"Okay," Jake said, "let's begin first with the ten episodes I said I would clear up."

"Start with Colorado," Steele urged. "Jake, how about Pueblo, Colorado?"

On the night of October 1, 1942, Jake confessed, he robbed an old woman of $47 and then choked her to death, after first clubbing her with a wrench. At Ogden, Utah, he recalled, while breaking into another house in the predawn hours he stabbed an old man to death while the victim was sound asleep in bed. Total net for the caper $3. "I don't know why I killed him," Jake said. "It just seemed like a good idea at the time." Next, South Bend, Indiana, 1942. Mid-October, day unknown, between 1 and 2 a.m.

"I had hooked up with a colored kid named Smith, about 27, and we'd burglarized some houses in South Bend," Jake remembered. "We didn't meet no opposition or nothing and we didn't do anything; that is, we didn't hurt nobody. So on this night we decided to hit this two-story house. We cut a hole through the backdoor screen, found the door unlocked and walked right in. There were two people, a man and a woman, sound asleep in the lower floor bedroom. I told my accomplice to kill them. I went upstairs to see what I could steal and, while prowling around, found a small boy fast asleep in the bedroom up there. I was armed with a piece of pipe and, not wanting to be discovered, I hit the boy across the head a couple of times, smashing his skull. The blow killed him instantly. Counting the two downstairs, that wiped out the family.

All we got for our troubles was a couple of pieces of cheap jewelry."

As Jake spilled his guts, Warden Smith suddenly stopped him. "Jake," he said, "we don't want you to be telling us that you did a lot of things or that you didn't do them. You might take credit for every unsolved murder in the United States."

Jake stiffened. How dare the warden question his integrity.

"I'm not making this up," Jake said. "You will just have to believe me."

"Okay, all right," the warden said. "Go on."

"Well, I have an interesting account from an investigator who wants to know if you killed a priest down out of Centralia, Missouri, in 1942."

"There is one thing you can go to bed with tonight and rest assured of, and that is I will never tell you that I done a crime that I haven't, or that I have an accomplice when I did not," Jake said.

"How about this priest in Missouri?" persisted the warden.

"Well," Jake said, "that is getting way off the course."

"Ever been in Centralia?"

"You see, every case you ask me about you think I am lying," Jake said.

"I don't think you're lying," the warden said. "I am asking you about this one. I am telling you a priest was killed and robbed in Centralia, Missouri, during the time you were not in prison."

"I said you might think I am lying. I meant that you might think I am lying about the statement I was going to make of meeting the father. When I say it you might think I am lying."

"How's that?"

"Well," Jake said, "I could say, 'Oh, yes, that was me, I killed him,' because I have been reading up on the case in detail from old files; in fact, every major case that has happened in the United States. Now, when you say about this priest being killed, I remember it well. I know the details."

"Were you in on that deal?" the warden asked.

"You will have to give me more time," Jake said.

"Let's get back to the original ten cases he agreed to discuss," Steele said.

"No," the warden said, "I am trying to get something here. Frankly, Jake, I'll be honest with you. I was cheating on you a little bit there. Actually, the priest wasn't killed in Centralia when you were serving time in Fort Madison. He was not one of your victims. But I am interested in what you did between the time you had that trouble with that prominent citizen in Benton Harbor and the time you got arrested there on the morning of October 23. I mean, did you kill somebody every night or just certain nights of the week that you felt like it."

"I wouldn't go so far as to say I killed somebody every night," Jake said.

"Did you carry a gun?"

"I never fooled with a gun. But some of my accomplices did."

"What kind of guns did they carry?"

"All kinds," Jake said. "Everything—38s, 45s, German Mausers."

"You never went much for guns yourself?"

"No, never."

"Ever take anything besides money?"

"When I was young, I did."

"Did you ever go for jewelry?"

"When we had a 'fence,' we went for anything—jewelry, dope, money."

"How about furs?"

"Them, too—when we had a 'fence'."

"Did you have an outlet for furs and jewelry?"

"Yes, in Chicago," Jake said. "There's always a 'fence' in Chicago."

"How about women, Jake?"

"Oh, a little bit," Jake said. "I was not much on women."

"Did you go out with the girls?"

"I fooled around with them somewhat, but not much. I ain't willing to waste too much money. I lost all mine gambling mostly."

"You never got into prostitution or pimping or that bracket of the trade?"

"No," Jake said, "I never believed in that."

"What did you do between the time you left Fort Madison and the time you showed up in the Chicago area?"

"Got a job," Jake said. "That was only for a couple of months. I was a pretty rough character. I'd done a little of everything."

"Tell us about those incidents in Omaha," Steele said.

"Well," Jake said, "one night I went out and I killed a man. The next night I killed two women. And the next night I beat this Stribling fellow up, and that I went to the penitentiary for."

"Did you get anything out of the house where you killed that man in Omaha?"

"Not a thing," Jake said.

"How did you get into that house?"

"Walked right through the back door."

"How many people appeared to live there?"

"Maybe two or three."

"Was the man the only one at home at the time?"

"Yes."

"What time of night was that?"

"You can believe this or not," Jake said, "but it was in the wide open daytime."

"What time of day?"

"Sunup."

"Sunup?"

"Yes."

"He was in bed?"

"Yes."

"Did he get out of bed?"

"No."

"You killed him in bed."

"Yes."

"What did you hit him with?"

"A hand axe I found in the house."

"How many times did you hit him?"

"Several times is all I remember."

"What did you do with the axe after you struck him?"

"Hid it in a pile of lumber behind the house."

"Did you take anything from the house?"

"Not a thing," Jake said. "I was not even looking."

"Did you rummage through the house at all?"

"I tell you I was not even looking for nothing, I don't know why I did it, I can't explain. You can call it what you want. Say I'm crazy or whatever you want, but as I recall, when I got arrested, I had around $50 on me, and they never even took a penny of it. They did not charge me with robbery. While I was there, a little girl came in and I managed to slip out without her even seeing me. All this happened in wide-open daytime. I walked right through the room she was in."

"Did you see the girl?"

"Sure," Jake said. "She was about 11 years old."

"Eleven years old?"

"Sitting near the bed reading a book. I walked right by her, walked right out the back door. Craziest thing."

"You said you got a job," Steele said. "With the paper company. Were you out murdering and carrying on these burglaries all that time?"

"Sure," Jake said. "That is all I was doing."

"That was a good dodge on that job," Steele said. "The job was just a dodge, then."

Jake said, "Working was a stall. We—my accomplices and me—were stealing every night."

"What did you do with all your loot?"

"Run all of it down at the Northshore and blew it, throwed it all away."

"In the crap joints?"

"Yes."

"What about those two women you killed? Why did you do it?"

"It started out as pure burglary," Jake said. "I got into the house through a basement window. The only weapon I had was a ballpeen hammer I'd stolen from another house. I did not find anything in the basement worth picking up so I went upstairs into the kitchen. Then I came out right by the front room and then over the side bedroom where a woman was sleeping and I killed her. A baby was asleep in a crib but I never touched it. I killed the woman, though, and then went upstairs and killed another woman in bed up there. She also had a kid with her, three or four years old, but I left the kid alone. Then I went outside and run."

"You did not harm either child?" Steele wanted to know.

"No."

"How old were the women you killed?"

"Young," Jake said. "Both were young."

"Where did you hit them?"

"Over the head."

"With this ballpeen hammer?"

"Yes."

"Did either woman scream?"

"No, they didn't know I was even in the house. Element of surprise."

"The children did not wake up?"

"The little boy did."

"The three-year old?"

"Yes."

"What did you do?"

"I picked him up and put him to bed in another room."

"Did he stay awake, did he scream or cry?"

"No, not a peep," Jake said. "He gave me no trouble at all."

"What did you do with the hammer?"

"Throwed it away on my way up the street to a place called the Dreamland Club, where I had a few drinks."

"Then what did you do?"

"I left the area that night," Jake recalled. "I went back to the Northside and got $75 and that is why the police did not push me very hard on them murders because they admitted when I came back that I had lots of money, and then one of the women's husbands admitted there was no money in the house, that I could not have gotten it from them. Therefore, they did not crowd me too much on the murders after they caught me in the Stribling affair."

"Jake," Steele said, "did you ever consider going straight?"

"Sure," Jake said. "I even got a job working for a coal company in Chicago. I was out there in the dark pitching coal at 4 o'clock in the morning at 8 below zero for $10, $16 and $18 a day. You know I would not have been doing that kind of slave labor if I had any intention in the world of stealing anything. I had actually decided to give up my old ways and live a good, clean life when, one night, I was walking down the street in Chicago and a police car pulled up alongside and throwed an automatic on me. I told 'em exactly who I was and everything, but they took me down to the station anyway; they did not have a thing on me, nothing, but then they found my prison discharge paper in my coat pocket and spent the next hour talking to me about it. Naturally I did not tell them I just got out of the penitentiary. If I told them that I would be sure to be bumped, but I told them I was working, where I had been that night, and they checked my story out and found I was telling the truth. Still they wouldn't let me go. They seemed to think I was up to some crime.

"Finally, one of the officers reached inside my coat pocket and pulled out No. 14314; that is, a letter from the prison with my number on it. That did it. They said, 'Book him.' Well, they hauled me down to the Bureau of Identification but they couldn't get nothing on me, so they took me to the Stock Yards Court and set my bail at some ridiculous figure I could not make, and then took me down to the house of detention for a trial. They kept me in the pen for three weeks—and still couldn't get nothing on me. Finally, they brought me back to court and fined me $1 and costs and no commitment.

"When they turned me loose, some officers went out ahead of me to the place where I boarded with these colored people and told everybody I had a prison record. So one fellow took me off to the side and told me I'd better leave. He said the police said they were coming out and pick me up every day or two. The cops also told them, 'That nigger killed three or four people.' Then I went to the office of the company I worked for and the man told me it was up to me whether or not I quit. The cops had told him the same story, and he told them, 'We don't give a damn how many people he's killed, just so he don't kill nobody here,' but the treatment I got from the fellows at work, I just couldn't take it, so I just pulled out. That was in January of 1942. I was going straight until then. I was really serious about giving up all that stealing and killing. But those goddamned cops in Chicago is what started me on the road back to crime."

Jake Bird's confessional at Walla Walla lasted for three days. He was verbose, always fencing, always reaching for time. Listening, Pat Steele had to wonder how much sadistic pleasure Jake got out of murdering another human being. He wanted to ask him, "How long can you go without cutting a throat?" and then answering his own questions, he could envision Jake's reply: "Sometimes, a long time." "You mean," Steele told himself, imagining the dialogue, "you have the urge under control? You can take it or leave it alone? You can cut two or three throats with a friend of an evening and then taper off by going home and only cutting one more before getting into bed?"

By now, Jake was front-page news across the country.

The papers played him up big. Sample, this from the *Chicago Tribune:*

Walla Walla Wash., Jan. 9—(AP)—Warden Tom Smith of the Washington State Prison announced late today that Jake Bird, condemned negro axe slayer, had said he could "clear up" 10 more slayings over the country, including the unsolved killing of Lillian Galvin and her maid in Chicago in 1942.

The 45-year-old black transient, sentenced to hang Jan. 16, asked for an attorney, the warden said.

The warden thereupon named attorney Charles Luce, of Walla Walla, to represent Bird. Luce joined Bird and prison officials in conferences at the prison.

Bird has already admitted complicity in 12 slayings over the U.S. the past 20 years.

Warden Smith emphasized that Bird did not say he committed the additional 10 killings, but only that he could clear them up.

In the Chicago case, Mrs. Lillian Galvin and her maid, Edna Sibilski, were killed Oct. 22, 1942, and $28,000 in jewelry and three fur coats valued at more than $3,000 were taken from their home, prison officials said.

Rewards totaling $16,000 were offered for solution of the case and nearly 1,000 persons questioned. Preliminary questioning today, Warden Smith said, showed that Bird was a three-hour drive away from the slaying scene the next day.

State's Attorney William J. Tuohy of Cook County, Ill., had called upon investigators to question Bird about the Galvin case.

Earlier today, W.L. Welch, South Bend, Ind., police officer, one of numerous officials from over the country here questioning Bird, said that Bird had given additional details about the slaying of a retired watchman, his wife and son there. He said Bird admitted a part in the crime.

A special investigator for the State of Iowa, Dwight Bender, also questioned Bird about the slaying of Jack Winfield at Davenport, Iowa. Bird had commented that authorities had the "wrong man" when shown a picture of the accused man in that case.

Upon his return to Tacoma, Pat Steele called Dr. Larson in and told him about his talks with Bird.

"Jake's singing like a bird," Steele said.

"But is it the *truth*?" Dr. Larson wanted to know.

"I believe him," Steele said. "He has nothing to lose getting it off his chest."

"For example?"

"Well," Steele said, "he told about the time in Cleveland. He was sitting in this tavern, making no bones about the fact he was flat broke. He needed some walking-around money. All he had in his pants pocket was 13¢. So he hit the street."

"Was that the time just after he got out of Utah State Prison? Rooming with a former convict?"

"Yes," Steele said. "They'd heard over the radio about a slasher who was always cutting up people in Cleveland. So, in April they decided to go up there and prowl some houses. They figured that if they got caught they'd just cut up some people, making it look like this crazy guy, the slasher, did it. So they rented a little shack and settled in for a lengthy period of prowling."

"Wait a minute," Dr. Larson said. "Did you tape what Jake told you?"

"Every bit of it," Steele said.

"May I read it?"

"Take it with you," Steele said. "But don't keep it for long. Governor Mon Wallgren is waiting to look at it."

"I'll bring it back tomorrow."

That night, Dr. Larson scanned the transcript. It confirmed what he had suspected about Jake Bird. Jake seemed to enjoy his work. In the transcript, Jake talked with great enthusiasm about the Cleveland capers:

"The first person we caught was a man," Jake said. "We nailed him in this little shack and robbed and beat him to death. No, I take that back. We did not beat him to death. We robbed him—and then we *stabbed* him to death. We cut his head off. I can't say just what part of the body I disposed of or which part my partner disposed of. I think he took the torso an' I got the legs. I took mine in a sack to a creek called Bull Run and pitched 'em in there; he throwed his here an' there; sometimes in an alley, all around."

According to the transcript, the victim was 40 years old. He was bald. Jake said it was the first time in his life he was fascinated by a bald head.

"The slashing took place in a very rundown, shabby part of Cleveland's colored district called Little Harlem," Jake said for the record. "We had a Dodge sedan and hauled the body to Bull Run Creek. The guy was white. We took $67 off him. He also had a pocket watch, but we refused to take it. We didn't want to get caught with it. We threw it into the creek.

"We then stripped the guy of his clothes. We burned them in the stove in his shack. A couple days later, when the papers came out, we saw plenty about the murder. Just as we figured, it was blamed on the Mad Killer, the guy we'd been reading so much about."

In the transcript, Steele had asked Bird what the weapon was he killed the man with. Bird said it had been a jackknife. Had the victim been stabbed in the head? Yes, Jake said, and then they sliced him up. He said they were very careful not to *hit* their victims, because that wasn't the way the Mad Killer worked. "Stabbing, cutting 'em up—*that* was his style," Jake told Steele. Pat wanted to know if his partner was still alive. Jake didn't know. "I'm the poorest man on names in the United States," Jake said. "All I know is that at the time he got out of prison he invited me to join him after I was released. The only name I had for him was Slim."

"Only Slim? Is that the only name you have for him?" Steele said.

"One night we put on this show at the penitentiary," Jake recalled. "The name of the play was 'Dan Chain Lightning.' This guy I'm tellin' you about played an old lady's part with a dress on. Everybody called him Slim There were only two or three blacks in the joint, so prison authorities should remember him easily."

Jake's Day in Court

BACK in Tacoma again, Pat Steele's face was haggard from the rigors of the Jake Bird interrogation. Across from his desk sat Dr. Larson.

"We have a strange one here, Charley," Pat said. "He never gives you a straight answer."

"I know what you mean," Dr. Larson said. "He talks a lot in bits and pieces."

"Yes," Pat said. "I went over there firmly convinced I had an inside track—that he would come clean."

"Don't let it get under your skin," Dr. Larson told him. "Listen to him closely. I believe that out of all Jake's verbiage you'll eventually be able to determine the truth."

"Jake never talks in sentences," Steele said. "He talks in whole paragraphs. Here, listen to this."

Steele had a copy of the transcript and he started to read:

> ME: Jake, what I am trying to get at is to put this last hour to good advantage for your own soul. Confession is good for the soul, as your preacher would say.

BIRD: You don't think I believe that, do you?

ME: Yes, I do. When you talk to the preacher, you're talking to the Lord through him.

BIRD: I say, do you *really* think I believe that?

ME: I think you do. You claim to be telling the truth.

BIRD: I am. Anybody else wouldn't even question it. You don't think I gotta spill my guts to you just to square myself with the Lord, do you? You sound like a preacher. Don't snow me, brother. I ain't got but one thing to do—that is, to tell you all I been saying is a lie—that I ain't signin' nothing—that I was just bluffin'—and then go in there to the chapel, get down on my knees an' ask God to forgive me. An' he'd forgive me, too. You cannot intercede in God's business. We gotta seek our own salvation. There's no use of a preacher fella tellin' me I gotta confess I kilt a man. But right is right. A little right don't hurt anybody.

ME: Why then, Jake, did you tell us about all those murders? What was your purpose?

BIRD: Because everybody is sayin' I ain't connected with them. That's the big reason I told you. I kilt those people—and a lot more."

"Then you're assuming that Jake is guilty of all those homicides?" Dr. Larson said.

"Guilty as sin," Steele said.

A couple of days after Dr. Larson and Pat Steele talked, Jake Bird was back on the front pages again:

Olympia, Wash., Jan. 12—(AP)—Attorneys for Jake Bird, transient who has admitted to the slaying of at least 12 persons, today filed papers with the State Supreme Court requesting:

1. A Writ of Habeas Corpus in the case Bird has an appeal pending.

2. If no appeal is pending, a Writ of Certiorari.

3. A restraining order preventing Warden Tom Smith from carrying out Bird's scheduled execution Friday morning.

The high court took no action on the petition today.

The petition, filed by John Tuttle of the Walla Walla law firm of Tuttle and Luce, said Bird allegedly wrote a letter from the penitentiary at Walla Walla to the Clerk of the Pierce County Court, purporting to appeal his conviction of slaying two Tacoma women.

It was not clear whether the letter arrived within the statutory time for making an appeal or whether it was a proper method of making an appeal.

If it were ruled that an appeal is pending as a result of the letter, Bird's execution would automatically be stayed until the appeal was disposed of.

If it were ruled that no appeal is pending, the attorneys request the high court for a Writ of Certiorari, which, if granted, would bring records in the case from the Pierce County Court to the Supreme Court for review to determine whether the purported appeal was good or not.

A copy of the action was served on Prosecutor Pat Steele this afternoon for the Walla Walla attorneys who say they entered the case "as an act of charity for a man who may have been deprived of important constitutional rights" and at the request of Warden Tom Smith.

On the morning of January 16, Bird got his stay of execution from Governor Wallgren. That night, instead of hanging at the end of a rope, he was accusing two Chicago prisoners by long distance telephone of participating with him in a double slaying.

Newspaper details of the hookup follow:

Walla Walla, Wash., Jan. 16—(AP)—Talkative Jake Bird, oft-times assuming a belligerent tone, charged two prisoners from Chicago by phone tonight of helping him kill two persons. He admonished one of the men curtly:

"I'm trying to get you to act right. If you don't shut up, you're going to get everyone hung."

An argumentative response from the accused man on the other end of the unprecedented long-distance hookup from the Washington State prison prompted the condemned axe slayer's sharp retort.

Bird, who was saved from hanging early today by a 60-day reprieve, reviewed many details of the killing of Mrs. Lillian Galvin and her maid in Evanston, Ill., in 1942. Acting Evanston Detective Chief Harry Engstrom directed prison arrangements for the unique chapter in the bloody Bird case, and the accused men were in the office of the Chicago *Herald-American.*

Bird told the two Chicago prisoners, identified as Lovell Boykins and William (Sugar Man) Hockett, to "tell the truth about the whole affair and make the best deal you can."

Bird talked first with the man identified as "Sugar Man" Hockett. He had told officers previously that "Sugar Man" was only 17 at the time the crime was committed and that he felt responsible for the youth.

Bird's opening words were:

"Hello, is that you, Sugar Man?"

On the other end of the line, Sugar Man denied knowing Bird or anything about the case. Bird argued with him, at times getting tough in his conversation.

Bird described the crime. He said that the two women were killed by Sugar Man and a man who is now serving time in the Michigan State prison on another murder charge. Bird then talked with the other man. "Lovell, this is Jake." Boykins had had no connection with the crime except going along with them and helping dispose of the loot, Bird said. "I got acquainted with you in your gambling joint," Bird told Lovell. "I just call you to tell you what happened that night and what you could do to help the situation. Your part wasn't very heavy—you got scared and ran."

A third man Bird also talked with was described as "Shaky Jake." Bird said that a brother-in-law of "Shaky Jake" had been given all the jewelry and furs from the Galvin robbery except for two pieces of jewelry. Frequently during the conversations in which he talked with each of the three men twice, Bird became argumentative, and occasionally profane. He pleaded with them to do what he thought was right. There were two sets of earphones used and all present took turns listening in. The three men at the

Chicago end seemed frightened and excited and occasionally stuttered.

Engstrom said he was convinced that one of the men on the Chicago end of the conversations would break down and confess. He said he was satisfied that a solution of the case had been obtained.

During most of the conversations, Bird asked leading questions, which the men in the Chicago jail were forced to answer.

After Governor Wallgren granted Bird a stay, the prisoner was returned to his cell at the Pierce County jail in Tacoma. There he drafted two trusties to type out his appeal documents and began bombarding the state Supreme Court. With boundless energy he kept dictating appeal briefs on an around-the-clock basis. He hammered away at the admission of one of the Tacoma police officers that he'd beaten him unmercifully on the night of the Kludt killings. What actually happened, claimed Bird, was that he was shoved into a patrol wagon and driven up and down the streets while the police kicked, punched and slugged him around "till my teeth flew like popcorn." When they finally got around to taking him to the County Hospital, he said, a doctor came out, looked at him and said, "Why, the bastard isn't *dead* yet," and went away.

Jake finally won his day in court. On May 20, 1948, he appeared before the state court after "firing" his court-appointed lawyers, Selden and Paulsen.

Dr. Larsen recalls the details: "Talk about bizarre appearances. Jake put on a show such as the solemn Temple of Justice chambers in Olympia had never seen—and probably never will see again. The handcuffs and leg irons, which had shackled him for the trip from the Pierce County jail to Olympia, had been removed before Jake entered the chambers. He then strolled in, took it slowly and coolly up the aisle. He was very confident, trim as a dancer, and he was dressed quite attractively in a brown, conservative suit, a white shirt, and a dark tie. The point of a maroon handkerchief protruded from his breast pocket.

"Special pains were taken to clarify the waiver-of-immunity business: That Jake had asked to make a statement, and that his statement there would subject him to the state's cross-examination; that questions would be asked and *had* to be answered; that anything he said could be held against him later. Did he understand all that? He did. 'All right,' he was told, 'then you may begin. And make it loud and clear.'

"Jake was armed with a score of law books. He'd borrowed them from the prison library in Walla Walla. Gesturing with both fists, kicking one foot and then the other, he shouted: 'Your Honors wantta know how the police got that confession outta me? They opened the cell door and they yelled at me, "Get in there, you black sonofabitch!" and he illustrated his words by swinging both fists and kicking the air. Then, he went on, "They yelled at me, "Get outta there, ya black bastard!" And again he feinted with a left hook, a right cross and a deft kick. 'Your Honors,' he told them, 'are going to ask why I committed that crime. But I ain't sayin' I committed that crime. Even if I did it, I'm entitled to a fair trial. I don't know nothin' about no habeas corpus or state ex rel, but I know about a fair trial. How do I know? 'Cause Warden Tom Smith told me so. And Warden Smith ain't lied to me yet.'"

The hearing lasted for a full hour. Afterward, Robert C. Cummings, who covers the political scene in Olympia for the *Tacoma News Tribune*, bumped into one of the Supreme Court judges, a close friend, as he was going home.

"That was quite a performance by Bird today," he said.

"Yes," agreed the judge. "But he talked too long."

"Too long?" Cummings said. "There's no time limit on appeals in a capital case."

"He still talked too long," the judge insisted.

"How so?"

"Well," the judge pointed out, "he described that room —the murder scene—which he said he'd never been in."

Jake Bird had unwittingly put a *hex* on himself!

Unlike conventional prisoners, condemned men are not subjected to a work routine; they can do with their time what they like—sleep all day, or, as was Bird's habit, read all night. He averaged a dozen books a week. His quenchless interest was restricted to one theme: law literature. He consumed hours each day leafing through law books, compiling research that he hoped would help reverse his conviction. This thirst soon depleted the shelves of the prison library.

Bird continued writing letters protesting his conviction and asking for a new trial. He charged that he had not had a fair trial. According to the way he figured it, the "hostile atmosphere" in Tacoma had made it impossible to empanel an unbiased jury, and therefore, a change of venue should have been granted.

But the bulkiest of Bird's claims was aimed at the arresting officers and his two defense attorneys, J. W. Selden and Arthur W. Paulsen. He insisted that the police had wrongfully beaten a confession out of him, forced him to sign an illegal statement; as for Selden and Paulsen, he shrugged them off as "incompetent and inadequate." Furthermore, he said, they had not prepared any real defense for him in the original trial, and this lack of effort, he implied, had been deliberate—an act of collusion between the defense and the prosecution.

These were grave assertions, reflecting upon the integrity of two respected lawyers and a distinguished judge.

Last Ditch Stand

ON May 23, 1949, four days before his latest appointment with the hangman was to be carried out, Jake was back in court. He had successfully won a hearing "on order to show cause in the matter of the application for a Writ of Habeas Corpus" before Judge Sam M. Driver, of the District Court of the United States for the Eastern District of Washington, Southern Division, at Walla Walla. There was no jury and Bird, at his own request, acted as his own counsel. C. John Newlands, assistant attorney general of the State of Washington, and Pat Steele represented the state.

This was the only known occasion that Jake Bird was ever on a witness stand and under oath.

The hearing, in part, went like this:

"Are you ready, Mr. Bird?" asked Judge Driver.

"Yes, sir, your Honor."

"Are you ready, Mr. Newlands?"

"Ready for respondent," Newlands said. "I might say, this case has recently gone through the courts of the State of Washington and the United States, being handled by the prosecutor's office of Pierce County, and I have asked them to asist me in this matter. Mr. Patrick M. Steele is the prosecuting attorney, and I have asked him to argue, and present some of the evidence in this case."

"Well," Judge Driver said, "he may be admitted for the purpose of appearing in this case. Mr. Bird, you are present here acting in your own behalf as petitioner without counsel. I might say that the Court did not appoint counsel; I'd like to have the record show that the court did not appoint counsel for Mr. Bird because it appeared from his petition there were no complex or difficult questions of fact which the Court felt it could pass upon without the aid of counsel so far as Mr. Bird is concerned. Now, I believe from reading your petition, Mr. Bird, that at least your principal contention is you were deprived of your rights under the federal constitution in your trial and conviction was brought about by a confession which you were forced to make, an involuntary confession, isn't that your principal point?"

Jake said, "Well, no, sir, your Honor, that is *one* of the principal points."

"What are the others?" Judge Driver wanted to know.

"The next principal point is that a fair hearing of the change of venue motion will convince this Court that a fair trial could not be had in Pierce County, and to put a man on trial in an atmosphere where he can't get a fair trial is denying him due process of law," Jake said.

"Yes," Judge Driver said, "I remember you had that point also."

"Okay," Jake said. "Now, the next point is, even the argument that I took to the State Supreme Court about the counsel would ordinarily solely be a state question. I understand fully that all it needed was that they appoint counsel that was a member of the bar and so forth, but in view of the fact what this man did, and the Judge forcing him on at a hearing that I wasn't present at, that in itself is saying that the State of Washington isn't enforcing the law."

"You mean on your appeal?" Judge Driver asked.

"No, at my trial," Jake said. "Now, on this appeal to the State Supreme Court, as this gentleman stated, he puts me in a little difficult position. The points I brought up to your Honor in this writ was the points that I'm fully prepared to prove. Now, if they wants to present any part of the record, your Honor, they can present all the record they want, because there's nothing in it but this so-called confession, and I can prove that."

"I merely want a statement of your points now," Judge Driver told him.

"Well," Jake said, "the statements of my points briefly is that I was arrested about 2:15 in the morning. I was taken. . . "

"Well, don't go over it in detail," Judge Driver said. "You claim that you were mistreated and beaten and forced to confess, and that confession was used in your trial?"

"Yes, sir."

"Another one is you were improperly denied a change of venue, and it was impossible for you to have a fair trial because of the inflamed condition of public opinion in Pierce County," Judge Driver said. "Now, what is another point?"

"That I paid for testimony I didn't get," replied Jake.

"I'm not concerned with your appeal at all," Judge Driver said. "All I'm concerned with is whether you had a fair trial in the Superior Court. If you had a fair trial, then I'm not concerned with whether or not your appeal was properly conducted; that's a matter for the Supreme Court of Washington to decide."

"Well," Jake said, "then my point is, in the Superior Court they beat this so-called confession out of me, that I did not have proper counsel . . ."

"Now, I don't quite understand that," Judge Driver said. "Was counsel appointed for you?"

"Counsel was appointed for me."

"Two lawyers?"

"Yes, sir."

"In what way do you claim that you weren't properly represented. Were they incompetent?"

"They was incompetent, and besides that they created so much adverse publicity, along with the prosecutor's office, that it deprived anybody of the possibility of thinking they was trying to conduct my defense. Further, they knew and had a list of witnesses that knew I had broken ribs, the skin beat off both my legs, several teeth knocked out, sprained back, and injured chest, they knew I had all this at the trial, and after having a doctor to examine me just three days before the trial, they didn't even call this doctor, but on the other hand . . ."

"They didn't call you either, did they?"

"No, sir."

"And that was because you had a number of prior felony convictions that they didn't want the jury to know about?"

"Well, that was the excuse, but my contention was to tell the jury about it."

"You wanted to testify, but your counsel decided it was best not to?"

"Yes," Jake said, 'but after all this, this counsel filed an affidavit to withdraw from the case. Now, your Honor, in talking to the jury, one counsel demanded an outright acquittal. He says, 'This man is not guilty of nothing—you seen him over in that alley an' you don't got a thing on him.' The other counsel says, 'We find ourselves in a difficult position. We have no legitimate argument to make for this man.'"

"Mr. Bird, I'm not inclined to go too deeply into the question of how good a job a lawyer in a state court did in defending an accused," Judge Driver said. "If I did that, I'd retry probably every case tried in state court, because every defendent convicted is dissatisfied with the way his lawyer handled the case, and I can't sit here and say such and such should have been smarter, should have used a better argument. I can't go into those questions. I must assume that attorneys appointed by the Court were capable and conscientious men. If one of your lawyers was incompetent and letting you down and actually trying to convict you, the judge would have replaced him in a minute; so where an attorney appointed by the Court conducts himself to the satisfaction of the Court, I must assume his services were such as at least not to violate the constitutional rights of the accused."

"But your Honor, the facts is on record. The attorney filed an application saying I had committed a dozen or more murders, and he didn't want the case," Jake said. "They go into court and argue this behind my back. If it's like your Honor says, if you assume this attorney wasn't going to do anything that would deprive me of getting a fair trial, then tell me, how could, after this attorney—why, that's a solemn..."

"I'd suggest you proceed to put on your proof, I think I understand your contention," Judge Driver said. "All I'm asking you to do now is tell me why you think I ought to release you on Writ of Habeas Corpus. I think I have that in mind. Now, proceed to put on your proof, your evidence, your testimony."

"Well, is the witnesses here?" Jake asked.

"I don't know," Judge Driver said. "You have yourself here, haven't you?"

"Yes, sir."

"All right, do you want to testify?"

"Yes, sir."

"All right, be sworn."

"Well, just a minute," Jake said, "there's some witnesses here I called, anyway."

"All right, if there are other witnesses, you may call them," Judge Driver said.

Jake looked around the courtroom and said, "I want to know is Officer Hickey here?"

"Apparently not," Judge Driver said.

"Well, in other words, it's not your duty to summon witnesses on a Writ of Habeas Corpus?" Jake asked.

"It's my duty to hear this case. I'm hearing it, Mr. Bird," Judge Driver replied. "You proceed with your proof, whatever you have here."

"Well," Jake said, "is Mr. Earl D. Mann here? Is Dr. Larson here?"

There was no response.

"Well," Jake said, "I guess you can see, now, that's just about the way it was in the courtroom. They testified to all this stuff in the courtroom, and now they are running away from me."

Whereupon John Newlands spoke up for the first time: "Your Honor, we have the certified copy of the transcript of the testimony taken by the reporter at the trial of the evidence of Dr. George L. Rickles; Officer Hickey, we have his testimony, and we have an extensive affidavit of Earl Mann, who was then deputy prosecuting attorney, who, of course, could not testify at the trial. So far there's just one man we haven't anything about."

"Well, now, your Honor, as I told you in that Writ, I didn't file that Writ for delay of any kind," Jake said. "I filed it because I know that Pat Steele and everybody that knows the case in Tacoma knows exactly what took place to Jake Bird, and they know, talking about what those people testified to, and all, and they was cross-examined. Now you get up on the stand, please, Mr. Steele, and I want to cross-examine you."

"But Mr. Bird," protested Judge Driver, "these men you asked to summon here are the very people you claim mistreated you."

"Absolutely."

"They testified at the trial that they didn't. What could you possibly hope to gain by bringing policemen here, who would testify to the same thing they did in your trial? Now, if you want to prove you were mistreated, the only way I can see, you'll have to testify, and then see whether I believe you or not."

"Well, just a second, please, Mister—your Honor, please."

"Yes, I think it would be better to say your Honor rather than Mister. Proceed."

"I made a mistake."

"All right."

"I've got two briefs missing," Jake continued, "but in one of those briefs, you asked me what I expect to prove by those witnesses that said after this young officer just out of the Navy lost his temper and struck me, that I got a single bit of abuse in that record. If your Honor hears this case, after I get through with Mr. Steele, I'll show you there is abuse from 2:15 until 11 o'clock, and I wish to question Mr. Steele now, if your Honor please."

"Mr. Steele?"

John Newlands explained, "He would like the prosecuting attorney to take the stand and be examined."

"Do you have any objection to that?" Judge Driver added.

"Not as long as Mr. Steele may still participate as assistant counsel here," Newlands said.

"Yes, he may have that privilege, of course," Judge Driver said.

For the first time, Pat Steele spoke: "If I can assist and establish something I will, your Honor."

"All right, proceed."

Pat Steele took the stand and Jake Bird began his direct examination.

"Will you state your name to the Court, please?" Jake said.

"Steele—Patrick M. Steele."

"And your occupation?"

"Prosecuting Attorney of Pierce County, Washington."

"And was you the prosecuting attorney along about October 30, 1947?"

"Of Pierce County, I was."

"And at that time you sent a deputy over to the county jail to take a confession from me, didn't you?"

"No, sir, I didn't."

"Well, one of your deputies did come over there, didn't he?"

"I was away on business in California. I learned about it later when I returned to Tacoma."

"My question, Mr. Steele, is did he come over?"

"I wasn't present when he came. I understand that he did."

"You understand that he did. And when you came back from California, he presented to you a so-called confession, or a confession, whichever you want to call it, didn't he?"

"There was available a writing which had been signed by Jake Bird and recounted the events of the night of October 30, 1947."

"And of course," Jake said, with a hint of sarcasm, "in this so-called confession you saw that I made those statements of my own free will and knew they could be used against me?"

"You mean," interrupted Judge Driver, "that was stated in the writing?"

"We have the confession here, if you want to examine it," offered Steele.

"Have I missed something?" John Newlands asked. "Is this concerning something at which Mr. Steele was personally present, or is he being asked to testify to something he knows his deputy did?"

"Mr Steele is being asked to testify was he the prosecuting attorney, and did he accept this as a confession and introduce it into the evidence, and what I'm solely trying to prove to Mr. Steele, and what I'm leading up to, your

Honor, is this: I'm leading up to show that Mr. Steele has said that the record don't show a single bit of abuse except Mr. Hickey's mistreatment, and I'm out to show that the record, according to Mr. Steele's own witnesses, does show other abuse."

"Is that a copy of the confession in your hand?" Judge Driver asked.

"Yes sir," replied Jake.

"I wonder if we shouldn't have it in here?" Judge Driver said, whereupon he asked for a pause in the hearing while the original confession was marked by the clerk and admitted in evidence as Respondent's Exhibit No. 1.

Finally, Jake went on with his direct examination.

"Mr. Steele," he said, "did you read this document that your deputy presented to you?"

"I have read it on several occasions."

"You've read this particular document?"

"That's right."

"And do you remember the statement, 'I make this statement because I want Mr. Mann and Mr. Lyons to have all the facts and the truth. I have not been mistreated by them, and no promises nor duress have been used to get me to make this statement. I know that this statement can be used against me.' Do you remember reading that statement?"

"I recollect there's something to that effect in there," Steele said.

"Mr. Bird," broke in Judge Driver, "I think that question is a little unfair, because as I understand, this witness wasn't present when the statement was taken, so he wouldn't have any occasion to advise you of your rights, would he?"

"But your Honor," Jake replied, "the confession shows —in other words, your Honor, here is the thing about it; now, I've been in this position ever since I've been fighting this case . . ."

"Well, now, let's talk about this particular document," Judge Driver said. "This man wasn't present when you signed it?"

"That's true," Jake said,

"All right, how could he advise you of your rights?"

"I'm out to show I was not advised of them at all," Jake explained.

"Well, if he knows about it, he can testify," Judge Driver said. "Mr. Steele, do you know whether he was informed of his rights before he signed the statement?"

"I have no personal knowledge, your Honor," Steele said. "As a matter of fact, I was not in the city, did not return until the following Monday."

"Well," Jake said," should I have been advised of my rights?"

"Oh, yes, yes, of course," Judge Driver said. "But that isn't a fact question."

"All right," Jake said. "Now, Mr. Steele, did you not say in your briefs and the various courts since we've been fighting this case, that my mistreatment by Officer Hickey in the patrol wagon was the only abuse that I could show?"

"In connection with what?"

"I object, your Honor," John Newlands said. "We have certain points in issue. One of them is the constitutional procedure which was followed in obtaining this confession. Now, I think Mr. Bird should confine his questions to the time of obtaining this confession, and not search through everything that has happened to Jake Bird since he was apprehended, for something to argue upon here. If he can pin his question down to the taking of this confession, and can show something was improperly done at the time of the confession, then I think this question could be proper, but not this general question."

"Well," Judge Driver said, "I think he should be permitted to show what has happened from the time of his arrest until his confession, because if a man is beaten and intimidated one night, and is afraid it would be repeated and subsequently signs a confession, obviously it would be involuntary, and he should be permitted to show what leads up to it. Mr. Bird, I'm allowing you more latitude than I would if you had an attorney, but I don't want you to go too far afield. What do you want to ask Mr. Steele next?"

"I'm trying to make it clear what I'm trying to bring out, that the record shows abuse from the time I was arrested up till the time I made the confession," Jake said.

"When you say the record, you mean the testimony at the trial?" Judge Driver asked.

"I mean the testimony at the trial, your Honor," Jake said. And then turning back to Pat Steele: "Now, Mr. Steele, you put an officer on the stand by the name of Mr. Hickey, didn't you?"

"That's right."

"And Mr. Hickey testified that he lost his temper in the patrol wagon and struck me several times, did he not?"

John Newlands leaped to his feet. "I object to that question," he said. "We're now not concerned with the confession. We do have the sworn testimony of Mr. Hickey which we can submit. I don't think Mr. Steele should be asked to answer that when we can present the testimony of Mr. Hickey."

"Do you have all that testimony?" Judge Driver inquired.

Steele answered for Newlands. "Your Honor," he said, "we have the direct, cross, redirect and recross."

Jack Bird was plainly flustered.

"These people are not trying to do nothing but cover up," he told the judge. "If I'm not supposed to show where that man beat me half to death . . ."

"Wait a minute, what you're asking is for this man to tell what somebody testified," Judge Driver said. "If we have the written testimony, that will be more reliable and more direct than for Mr. Steele to tell it from memory."

"I can say at this time my objections are not designed to keep Mr. Steele from admitting any evidence which is in issue, and I will relax my objection on that point," John Newlands said. "But I want to keep this from getting into a circus."

"Your Honor," Jake said, "the only circus that they are afraid is going to take place . . ."

"Let's just keep on the track here," Judge Driver said.

". . . is that I'll bring out that I was abused for eight hours, as I claimed," Jake continued.

"Well, you can very easily bring that out by taking the stand and testifying," Judge Driver told him, "and you can tell just exactly what happened to you."

"Your Honor, please, I would like to ask you one question for advice, if you'll advise me on that score," Jake said. "If those people beat me up and abuse me and force me to sign a confession, is that confession any good?"

"No, it's not, but that's the very question we're inquiring into," Judge Driver said. "I want you to *prove* that."

"I'll prove it," Jake said.

After more questioning of Pat Steele, then cross examination by John Newlands, and finally redirect examination by Jake, Steele was excused.

Jake looked up at Judge Driver.

"Your Honor," he said, "I wish to take the stand, please."

"All right."

"Shall I ask myself questions?" Jake wanted to know.

"No, you just tell your story in your own way," Judge Driver instructed him.

"Well," Jake began, "my name is Jake Bird, and I'm an inmate of the Washington State Penitentiary. I brought a Writ before this Court that said I was mistreated and abused. At the trial the state put an officer on the stand by the name of John Hickey to testify that he lost his temper in the patrol wagon, and that he beat me, and after he beat me that he snapped out of it in disgust and took a seat in the back of the patrol wagon. Now, this officer testified further that he didn't think Jake Bird was a man, he considered him a beast. He wouldn't say Jake Bird was severely injured, even though Jake Bird was lying on the sidewalk at the time. He further testified that he took Jake Bird to a hospital, and a nurse came out and looked at Jake Bird and said Jake Bird don't look so bad and they hauled him away without treatment."

"You mean Officer Hickey?" Judge Driver asked.

"Officer Hickey," Jake said. "He further testified that Officer Skattum was needed back at the scene, was the reason they hauled me away without treatment. He further went on to say that there was Officer Skattum, himself and the driver, and that I was handcuffed at the time of the attack. He says he didn't care where he hit me. He says he didn't count the blows that he struck. In other words, he says at the time he attacked me he wasn't thinking. Now, the only other question after this, he says I told him that Leroy did it. He asked me did I commit the crime, and I told him that LeRoy did it, and he says I said I was looking at the house."

Jake paused, took a deep breath, continued.

"Now," he said, "the state's main contention in fighting me all the way up to the United States Supreme Court is, look at the four witnesses' testimony about this so-called confession. Well, here is their testimony. Hickey says I said LeRoy did it. Lyons said I told him it was light in the house, and I could see, and that I had an axe an that I did it. Dr. Wright said it was dark in there, and when I went in there I didn't know what I had anyway. When I was taken to the county jail they got Sig Kittleson to say I went in the room and killed them. In this confession they say I was talking to another person and grabbed them, until the State Supreme Court asked Mr. Steele, 'What are you going to do about these four versions?' I want to know what makes their four versions so important. I'm not trying to get you confused, your Honor, because these are four direct controversions that can be nothing but lies, they cannot be the truth: it happened one way or the other if I did it. Now they've got *five* versions."

"Please the Court," John Newlands pointed out, "we're arguing the case now. I'd like to get just the facts before the Court now."

"Yes," agreed Judge Driver, "what you're on the stand for, Mr. Bird, is the purpose of testifying what you know about this case."

"Well, I'm telling you what I know about it," Jake said.

"You're arguing about what somebody else said, and what the Supreme Court did and so on," Judge Driver said. "That's argument. You're supposed to tell me what happened to you."

"Well, what happened to me was this. After Officer Hickey says that he beat me up at 2:15 in the morning, he says he hauled me to the hospital . . ."

"You're discussing again something that's in this testimony here," Judge Driver said.

"Yes, sir."

"That isn't anything you know about. You're on the stand to tell what you know about this. What did they do to you? You claim they forced you to confess. How did they do that? You may argue afterward. I'll give you a reasonable time to argue from this record and from circumstances and what somebody else said, but now you're on the stand for the purpose of testifying. You've seen trials enough."

"Yes, sir I've seen trials enough, but none like these."

"All right, go ahead."

"The point I can't get clear, I told you in my Writ that the record was reeking with perjury. Now, if we're going to take what those officers testified at the trial and try to say that those officers testified to the facts as they were, we're admitting it's been testified to . . ."

"You're arguing again, Mr. Bird. That isn't testimony," Judge Driver reminded him.

"Well, my testimony is this. I'm going to show you where I got other abuse that night.

"After Mr. Hickey took me to the hospital and hauled me to the Kludt home three times, they proceeded to the police station with me."

"Where were you arrested?" Judge Driver wanted to know.

"Out in an alley, a backyard, about a half-block from the Kludt home, on the other side of the street."

"One of the officers chased you?"

"No, sir, he was on his way to the home, and said, 'There's a man over in the alley.' They made up the story because they thought that justice was going to catch up with the so-called confession."

"They knew when they arrested you that they were going to force you to confess?"

"No, when they arrested me, they said they had a call to go to the Kludt home."

"Well," Judge Driver said, "what I'm trying to do is get an orderly sequence of your story. I want to get you started, if I can, so that you'll keep off of all this stuff that isn't doing you any good or me either. You were arrested a block from the home?"

"Yes, sir."

"All right, then what happened."

"Well," Jake continued, "they took me to the Kludt home, they took me to the hospital, they brought me back to the Kludt home..."

"Why did they take you to the hospital?" Judge Driver asked.

"Because I was severely wounded."

"How did you get wounded?"

"I got wounded when they took me to the Kludt home the first time, right after my arrest," Jake said. "Officer Hickey went into the house an came out and got in the patrol wagon with me, along with Officer Skattum, and he said, 'Nigger, you killed two white women!' I said, 'I haven't killed anybody.' He said, 'Well, who did it?' And I said, 'I don't know.' He said, 'Anybody else out here with you?' I said, 'Yes.' He said, 'Who is it?' I said, 'LeRoy.' He asked, 'Where's LeRoy now?' I said, 'With all this shooting and running around, where do you think he is?' He said, 'Did LeRoy go in the house?' I said, 'I don't know. I seen somebody come out of the back door and throw something away that looked like him.' He said, 'You're not sure that LeRoy committed the crime?' I said, 'No.' He said, 'You black sonofabitch, you're going to show me that LeRoy is down in the poolhall someplace, there's no LeRoy here!' And then he said, 'You're going to tell me about killing these women right now,' and he busted me across the bridge of the nose, and that's where I lay in the patrol wagon until they took me to the hospital on the second trip. No, they proceeded to the police station after taking me to the Kludt home three times and the hospital twice. They testified at the trial that I said when I was brought into the station..."

Judge Driver said, "I'm interested only in what actually happened and what you said, and not what they said, not what you said they said at the trial. The record will show what they said. I want to know what happened from your standpoint. Go ahead."

"Well," Jake said, "they took me to the police station, and they said I said at the station, 'Yes, I did.' They said they asked me did I do it, and I said, 'Yes, I did.' They said I asked for water and rest."

"But you didn't say yes, you did it, or did you, at the police station?"

"You want to know whether I said, 'Yes, I did it,' is that it?"

"Yes."

"Yes, sir, I said, 'Yes, I did it,' but I said I did it only because they done tortured me and put all manner of torture to me, and I had to say yes or get killed. I told them I wouldn't sign anything, and when I told them that, they proceeded to beat me some more. Then they gave me some water and said I had two hours of rest coming and took me to a cell. By now I had four teeth knocked out, I had my top lip cut clear through on both sides, I had several stitches in my head and face, I had my ribs cracked, and skin beaten off both legs down to my feet, and the scars is here today if you want to see them. That's the condition I was in. I rested from 5 o'clock till 7:45 and then was ordered back to the hospital."

"How long were you at the hospital?" Judge Driver asked.

"About an hour."

"And then where did they take you?"

"Back to the detective bureau making this confession," Jake said. "Lt. Lyons was there, and then in walked some officer who said, 'There's the damn nigger that killed the white women and raped one of them's dead body,' but still there's no other abuse in the record, according to them. The record shows what they did, and what happened is Jake Bird never had one wink of sleep from the time they arrested me until the time this so-called confession was made."

"How much time elapsed in between?" Judge Driver said.

"Well, 2 o'clock in the morning until 11 the next day."

"Was that the time you signed this confession?"

"Yes."

After more sparring around, during which Jake repeated how he had been cuffed around on the night of his arrest, Judge Driver asked, "Mr. Bird, how long was the trial after your arrest?"

"Twenty-four days, even though I was still wounded."

"Do you have any further testimony as to what happened there that you want to tell the Court, anything else you want to tell about what happened to you?" Judge Driver asked.

Jake shook his head.

"No," he said. "That's what happened to me."

"I see," Judge Driver said. He turned to John Newlands and said, "All right, cross examination."

"How old are you, Mr. Bird?" Newlands asked.

"Forty-seven," Jake replied.

"Where were you born?"

"Louisiana."

"When?"

"December 14, 1901."

"How long did you live in Louisiana?"

"Oh, about 20 years."

"Then where did you go?"

Impatiently, Jake suddenly turned to the judge and asked, "Has I got a right to object to it?"

"Yes, you have a right to object," Judge Driver said. "I think, though, he has a right to ask it; rather broad limitation in a case of this kind. Go ahead, you may answer if you can."

"Well," Jake muttered, "I just simply can't see how an immaterial thing like that matters, yet every question I asked off the record to prove my point, it don't matter. I don't know where I went from there, I can't truthfully say. I went somewhere, I just don't know."

"Did you go to school in Louisiana?" Newlands asked.

"Yes."

"What was the town you lived in?"

"It wasn't much of a town, just a place out in the country."

"It was a country school?"

"The nearest place was called Plummer," Jake recalled.

"How many years of schooling did you have?"

"I started when I was six and quit at 18," Jake said. "That would be about 12 years of school, I guess."

"And after that you worked?"

"If I may," Jake said, "I'd like to add a little something to that."

"All right, surely," Judge Driver said.

"Well," Jake said, "at that time they was giving school three months a year to colored people, and we had to walk about four or five miles to and from school every day, so you didn't learn very much."

"Then you went to work after you got out of school?"

"Yes. I was working before I got out of school."

"What kind of work?"

"Oh," Jake said, "I waited table, and common labor, just practically anything I could do."

"That was in Louisiana?"

"Well, some of it, and wherever I was and got a job."

"Where were you? Where did you go after you left Louisiana?"

"I went to New York, I went to Maine, I went to Boston, I went to Philadelphia, I went to St. Louis."

"Did you live in those places, or just visit them?"

"Well," Jake said, "I was there and didn't die. I lived everywhere."

"Did you work there?"

"Oh, I works a little bit some places, some places I didn't."

"Have you ever been convicted of any crimes before?"

"I object to that as immaterial," Jake said.

Judge Driver said, "You may show a prior conviction of felony only in this court, to affect the credibility of the witness."

Newlands said to Jake, "Have you ever been convicted of any felonies in any courts in the United States before?"

"Yes," Jake said.

"Where? Any in Illinois?"

"I think the record is plain on that," Jake said, evading the question.

"Well, this record isn't plain," Judge Driver said. "When a witness takes the witness stand, it may be shown if he has been convicted of felonies, and what the offense was."

Newlands asked, "Were you ever convicted in courts of the State of Utah?"

"Yes."

"Of what crime?"

Jake turned to Judge Driver. "Your Honor," he pleaded, "I again object to that as immaterial."

"Overruled," Judge Driver said.

"The objection is overruled," Newlands said. "Will you answer the question?"

"Do you want me to tell what crime it was?" Jake asked.

"Yes," Judge Driver said.

"Second degree burglary," Jake said.

"Were you ever convicted in the State of Iowa?"

"I was."

"Of what crime?"

"I object to that as immaterial," Jake said.

"Overruled," spoke up Judge Driver. "Mr. Bird, I might say that the only purpose of this, if you had taken the stand in your trial in Tacoma, these very questions would have been asked you. The theory is, when any witness takes the stand, whether he's the accused or not, it may be shown that he's been convicted of a felony, and that's in order to determine what weight should be given to his testimony. It goes to his credibility, and they may show that you've been convicted of felonies, and what the offense was; not any of the circumstances, of course."

Jake asked, "Now that I am on the stand is it proper for me to make a statement to your Honor?"

"I think it would be more orderly if you answer counsel's question, and then you will be permitted to testify again in rebuttal," Judge Driver said.

"The point is," Jake told him, "I wanted to ask your Honor about a particular question."

"All right."

"In order to aid me, you must remember I'm alone, I haven't got counsel. You said I've been around and in courts quite a lot. Well, all the courts I've been in ruled that it didn't make any difference what a defendent has been convicted of, all they may show is he's been convicted of a felony."

"That is the rule in some courts," Judge Driver said, "but my ruling has been in order to know what effect to give to a conviction it's necessary for a trier of the facts to know what the difference was. If a man is convicted of perjury, that would very vitally affect his credibility. If he had been convicted of something else, a crime of violence or lost his temper and hit somebody, that wouldn't affect his credibility very much, so my ruling has been and will continue to be, until I am reversed, that the felony may be shown, and what the offenses were."

"Well, then," Jake said, "I was convicted of assault and attempt to commit murder."

"Were you ever convicted in the courts of the State of Michigan?" Newlands pressed on.

"Yes," Jake said.

"Of what crime?"

"Of..."

"Was it burglary?"

"They have a new name for it there," Jake said. "It was only an attempt, the crime wasn't carried out."

"Did it correspond with the crime of burglary in the State of Washington?"

"I think so," Jake said. "In fact, just a second, I told you I was convicted in all those places, didn't I?"

"Yes."

"Well, that's a little bit wrong. I pleaded guilty in two cases and was convicted in the assault and attempt-to-commit murder case."

"Well," Judge Driver said, "I think the term 'convicted' would cover either a plea of guilty or finding of guilty by the jury or the court."

"Now, Mr. Bird," went on Newlands, "when did you come to the State of Washington?"

"October 27, 1947."

"That was three days before the offense of which you were convicted?"

"Yes, sir."

"Where did you enter the state?"

"I beg your pardon?"

"Into what city did you come? Did you come in through Vancouver, Spokane—how did you come into the state?"

"Oh, well, the first city I stopped at was Spokane, I think."

"And you came directly to Tacoma?"

"No, I think I came to Seattle first."

"What were you doing there?"

"What was I doing?"

"Yes."

"Well, I didn't have very much time to do anything. I just got there."

"Were you on a trip, a vacation, what were you doing? Were you looking for work?"

"Well, I just quit work, so if I got another job I would have certainly wanted to work."

"Now on the night of October 30, 1947, at 2 a.m., you state that the officers saw you climbing over a fence into the alley, is that correct?"

"No, sir, that is not."

"When did the officers first see you?"

"When I was standing up in an alley across the street from the Kludt home."

"Were you just standing there?"

"Yes."

"Did you have a gun on you?"

"No."

"Did you have a knife?"

"Sure, I did."

"The officers saw you?"

"Yes."

"What did you do then?"

"Nothing, until they said, 'Let's see what this man done over in the alley.'"

"You just stood there and waited for them?"

"No."

"Did you run?"

"No."

"Did you hide?"

"No, I didn't have a chance to hide."

"You saw them first, you said. Why didn't you stay there?"

Jake was growing flustered.

"Well, listen, you say..." he stammered.

"You were either running or hiding or standing there waiting," Newlands said.

Jake turned to Judge Driver once more. "Your Honor," he complained, "nobody is going to give me a chance to prove my case. I never committed that crime, that's the reason I didn't run. If I had been, the officers never would have seen me."

"Were you running, then?" Newlands asked.

"No, sir."

"Were you standing there?"

"I was standing there, just like I'm sitting here."

"Was this in the alley?"

"Yes, sir."

"Were you carrying an axe?"

"An axe?"

"What about a knife?"

"Don't you want to know about the axe?"

"All right," Newlands said, "what about the axe? Did you have an axe with you? You said you didn't have a gun, did you have a knife? Did you have the axe?"

"Mr. Newlands," Judge Driver said, "he said he had a knife, but he hasn't answered about the axe."

"Oh, your Honor," Jake said, "who would be standing in the alley with an axe? No, I never had no axe."

"When the officers came toward you, what did you do with your knife?"

"It was in my pocket."

"When did you take it out?"

"When Officer Sabutis said you is a—I should tell what he said—*black nigger.*"

"Were they trying to arrest you?"

"Absolutely."

"And you resisted?"

"I'd resist you right now if you walked up an said that."

"Why did you resist them?"

"Because he said, 'You is a black dirty nigger bastard, and if I'd known it, I'd have shot you down,' and I told him, 'I'll give you a chance to shoot me down now.' Had he not called me that, nobody would have got hurt."

"Did you attempt to cut the officers with your knife?"

"No, I didn't."

"What did you take the knife out for, then? Didn't you attempt to cut both of them?"

"No, I didn't attempt to cut them; I cut both of them. I cut Sabutis in the fight. The other one ran up and struck at me, and I threw my hand up, and he cut his arm, but I wish to add right here . . ."

"How did you lose your teeth?" cut in Newlands.

"In the patrol wagon, when Hickey and Skattum and all those people knocked them out."

"Going back to the knife," Newlands said, "what happened to it? Did the officers take it away from you?"

"Your Honor," Jake said, "is he proceeding legally?"

"Well, yes, Mr. Bird," Judge Driver said, "You can answer that, can't you?"

"All right," Jake said, "I throwed it down on the ground."

"Mr. Bird," Judge Driver said, "why do you think he isn't proceeding legally?"

"Well, simply this, your Honor. I cannot see, now, I put

in a Writ of Habeas Corpus, and I put down the witnesses I want called, and I solemnly swear that I haven't got money to prosecute this Writ . . ."

"Now you're on the witness stand as a witness, and he has a right to cross-examine you," Judge Driver said.

"Well, your Honor," Jake said, "I just want to know if he's proceeding legally."

"It's perfectly legal cross examination," Judge Driver said.

"I threw it down on the ground," Jake said.

"Was that after you cut the officers?"

"Yes."

"Where did Sabutis get cut? Did you stab him in the back?"

"I don't know where I stabbed him," Jake said. "All I know is when he run up and said what he did, that me and him got fighting. They said I had him around the neck and had him bent over there, what Sabutis said up on the stand at my trial. I'm telling you what happened. All I know, Sabutis said what he said and I took a knife and swung at him. What position he got in, or whether my knife went around his neck or not, or hit him in the face, all I know, he said what he said, and I said, 'If you feel that way, I'll give you a chance to kill me right now.'"

"Where did they take you in the patrol wagon?"

"Took me to the Kludt home, then to the hospital. I stayed in the wagon and a doctor came out and looked at me and said, 'He's not dead yet.' Then we went back to the Kludt home."

"Officer Hickey and this other officer were in the wagon with you?"

"Part of the time. You see, they'd stop all along the street and take relays."

"Your first contact with Officer Hickey was when you were put into the patrol wagon?"

"Well, I don't know," Jake said. "It seems to me that two officers came back where I was sitting and handcuffed me. Now, whether Officer Hickey was one of them, I can't truthfully say, but the first time I remember coming into any direct contact with him was when he started out to the Kludt home. He cuffed me around good. He'd exhaust himself and then let another one come in and exhaust himself."

"At the hospital, what did the doctor do for you?"

"He put stitches in my lips and stitches in my head and bandages on my leg. He told me it's best not to disturb the ribs, because if I'd bust them out of place, they didn't do anything to that, and he said the back would be all right, and the chest would be all right, so they bandaged my legs and stitched my head and lips."

"When you got back to the police station from the hospital, what did you do then?"

"About three or four uniformed officers took me over in a little dining room and asked me was I ready to confess, so I told them yes, an they told me to give them briefly what happened. When I told them this fellow was with me and he might have done it, they knocked me down in there and kicked and stomped me and kicked the skin."

"That wasn't the occasion, then, that you dictated this confession you signed?"

"I don't want that in the record no way. I didn't dictate nothing. Deputy Prosecutor Mann dictated it."

"Was that the time that you made a statement?"

"No, sir, that's the time they asked me questions, an after each question Earl Mann would tell the reporter what to write. I'd sit there and say yes, or no, or shake my head, an they dictated what they wanted to write."

"And that is the confession that we have before us now as it was typed out, that is the same confession that you say Mr. Mann asked you questions and you answered, and it was written out, and that's the confession you signed?"

"Yes."

"No further questions, your Honor," Newlands said.

Judge Driver stared down at Jake. He had some questions of his own he wanted answered.

"Mr. Bird," he said, "were some changes made in the confession after it was written out?"

"Yes, sir."

"Did you initial the changes that were made?"

"Yes, sir."

"Were they made at your request?"

"No, sir. They were made when they was reading the confession over, and said that I said in two places where I took money out of the purse, and asked me which one was correct, and I said either one, to suit your taste, so they initialed them out and told me to put 'J.B.' there."

Judge Driver had a copy of the confession in front of him, and he said, "Well, they lined it out, but this is your handwriting there, the 'J.B.' where you initialed it?"

"Yes, sir."

"All right, that's all then."

It was now time for redirect testimony and Jake went back to attacking his two lawyers who had defended him at his trial. Judge Driver had read excerpts of the testimony and he said it seemed to him that both Selden and Paulsen had fought hard for Jake, especially Selden.

"Did Mr. Selden continue to do that throughout the trial?" Judge Driver wanted to know.

"Well," Jake said, "he made objections and exceptions. I think I said that in the record it was littered with objections and exceptions."

"I thought you made some point that you didn't have effective representation by counsel," Judge Driver said.

"Well, do you want me to tell you that in my own way?"

"All right."

"I said it was a constitutional right for me to be represented by counsel," Jake said. "I said that this court nor no other court can say fairly, and I say so without trying to insult anyone, if anybody says a lawyer can go into court, and one lawyer get up and demand an outright acquittal, and the other one tell both judge and jury, 'You go ahead and hang that man, he should be obliterated.' What was that but a farce and a circus? That's no trial at all, despite all the records. I don't think they've got that in there."

"You mean one of your lawyers actually asked the jury to find you guilty?" Judge Driver asked.

"Well, he didn't say so in so many words," Jake replied, "but I'll tell the Court what he said, in so many words. He said, 'We find ourselves in a difficult position. It is our time to put in argument, and I know of no legitimate argument to make, and that there was evidence put in against this man that shouldn't have gone in the record, and there was evidence the state should have produced here that the state didn't produce; however, you find him guilty of anything you want to, that's all right with us,' speaking for both of them. Later, when we got before the judge, one argued for an hour, at least, for a new trial. After he sat down, the second one got up and told the judge I should be obliterated, that he had a motion before him for a new trial, but he was not going to put himself in a position to argue it. And so, your Honor, where was I truly represented by counsel, when this man filed a big affidavit in Court to quit the case just 12 days before my trial? He did this behind my back, but the judge forced him to stay on the case to protect my rights, and yet I never seen him no more until the case come up in court. Now, what kind of counsel is that? I say I was not properly represented by counsel. The same thing with the records. The state wasn't in a position to deny me the records, because, your Honor, you know it's a joke, where a judge can sit up an say, 'It's within my discretion,' but they didn't give me the record I paid for . . ."

"Well, that is not a matter for testimony here, Judge Driver said. "You're getting off into argument."

"But I'm getting into argument because I come in as a pauper to prosecute the Writ," Jake pointed out.

"All right, now, that's enough, unless you have some testimony," Judge Driver told him.

"I'm ready to submit my evidence if he's through putting in his evidence," John Newlands said.

"Mr. Bird, you're arguing from the witness chair," Judge Driver said. "Of course, I've told you not to do that, but you keep on doing it. If that's all the testimony, you may retire here."

"Could I say something after I step down," Jake said, "or do I have to quit now until they get through?"

"You will be permitted to argue when it comes time for argument, Mr. Bird. Now, step down."

After Newlands had finished submitting a number of documents as his "controverting evidence" to the Court, including evidence that Jake's application to the U.S. Supreme Court for certiorari was denied, Judge Driver asked Jake: "Do you have anything else to offer, Mr. Bird, other than argument now, I mean? I'm going to give you a chance to argue, of course."

"I asked you could I call Mr. Steele again, and you ignored me," replied Jake.

"Your Honor," Newlands said, "Mr. Steele does not feel anything can be gained by getting on the stand again. If the Court desires it again, we'll be glad . . ."

"Just a minute, your Honor, this man sitting here . . .," pointing to Pat Steele.

"What do you want to prove by Mr. Steele?" Judge Driver asked. "I'm not interested in any hot arguments between you and counsel."

"I'm not either, but I can't understand no such proceeding," Jake said.

"What do you want to prove by Mr. Steele?" Judge Driver asked. "You can understand the English language."

"I wants to question him about did he say the law

requires all the circumstances to be given to the jury about a man's mistreatment."

"You want to ask him if the law requires all the circumstances of mistreatment to be given to a jury?"

"Yes."

"Well, that isn't proper cross examination," Judge Driver told him. "That's a question of law. Just because he's a lawyer, you can't call him and ask him what the law is on a question like that. That isn't anything that would help you out."

"In other words," Jake said, "he don't know how to enforce the law as a prosecutor."

"I don't care whether he knows any law, or knows it all. The question we're inquiring into is a question of fact, whether your confession was voluntary or whether it was coerced, and Mr. Steele's idea of what the law might require as to putting facts before a jury has no bearing on that question that's helpful at all. Now, is there anything else you want to prove by him?"

"Well, it seems I have a chance to prove nothing. I can't prove . . ."

"Well, all right, let's put it this way," Judge Driver said. "The Court will take judicial notice of what you're attempting to prove by Mr. Steele. I'll take judicial notice that the circumstances surrounding a confession should be disclosed to a jury when a confession is put in evidence. Now, I'm assuming it's correct, what you're trying to prove by Mr. Steele. Now, do you have anything else to offer?"

"Well, if you'll take judicial notice of that, that's sufficient to me," Jake said.

"All right," Judge Driver said. "Now, do you have anything else?"

"Why, no, sir, I can't call no single witness I asked for. They're not here, and I'm a pauper, I haven't got a penny."

"The officers you wish to call are the police officers whose testimony is in evidence here in the record for your use and for my consideration," Judge Driver told him. "The Court didn't consider it necessary to bring them over here from Tacoma again for this hearing at somebody's expense, since we have the testimony already. If that's all the testimony, we can proceed with the argument, and I'll allow counsel for the respondent here a half an hour, and allow the petitioner an hour for argument. Because of his not being an attorney and the others being attorneys, I'll give him twice as much time as they. Can you cover the subject in half an hour?"

"Yes, your Honor," Newlands replied, "that's satisfactory with us."

"And you, Mr. Bird, would you prefer to argue first and then reply to them, or how would you like to use your time? Would you rather they'd go ahead first?"

"To tell the truth," Jake said, "I can't argue in an hour. I come down to prove a case, so if you simply want to shut it off and not hear the case . . ."

"How much time would you like to argue?"

"I come down here to argue what I intend to prove."

"Well, how much time do you want to argue?"

"Well, I certainly wouldn't impose on you."

"I think that an hour is ample time. I've considered what the issues are. These gentlemen can argue in a half an hour, you should be able to argue in an hour. The Court has already read all the testimony. I read the new testimony during the lunch hour. It's about two inches thick that you submitted with your petition, and then the exhibit put in evidence here, and it isn't necessary to read that over to me again. All you have to do is comment on the various things and what the Court should consider in connection with it."

"That's true enough, your Honor, but now your line of talk up there is just the same as every judge I've been before," Jake said.

"I don't care to hear that, Mr. Bird, but I'll let you

argue. Even though you are in your present situation, I'm not going to let you stand there and lecture me about what my duties are."

"I'm not lecuring," Jake said. "I'm lecturing that I've got no help, no lawyer."

"I know you haven't. If you want to take advantage of that and argue, all right. If you don't, we'll close the hearing right now."

"Naturally, I want to argue the hour. I still protest that isn't enough."

"The petitioner protests that an hour is not sufficient time to argue his case, and exception is allowed in the record. Proceed," ordered Judge Driver.

"I'm sorry that the Court thinks that I tried to lecture the Court and tell the Court its duties," began Jake.

"Well," Judge Driver said, "I think you're trying to put on a little show here, Mr. Bird, and I think we'll both get along better if we just stick to the issues."

"No, sir, I'm only trying to apologize. I'm sorry if my manner caused you to make that statement."

"Oh, I see. Well, that's all right."

"And I feel bad about it. That's why I brought that up."

"Your apology is accepted. That's quite all right. Proceed."

Whereupon, Jake presented his opening argument to the Court, then Pat Steele presented his argument to the Court on behalf of the respondent and, finally Jake presented his final argument.

In handing down his decision, Judge Driver pointed out that as in so many cases that came before his Court, the Jake Bird case originated and was prosecuted entirely in the state court. Jake was prosecuted for violation of the laws of the State of Washington, namely murder. He had been tried with the benefit of two lawyers appointed by the Court to assist him before a jury. The jury had found him guilty, and it was appealed to the Supreme Court and was before the Supreme Court of the State three times. It was also before the Supreme Court of the United States on petition of certiorari and on petition for rehearing.

"I mention all that merely to point out that it's a very heavy responsibility that this Court has in cases of this kind, particularly where there's a serious offense committed," Judge Driver said. "I have no power to grant this man a new trial. I can't send him back to Pierce County to be tried again. The only alternative I have is to deny his petition or order his release unconditionally from the penitentiary where he's in custody, and that being the case it's not only a rule of law but common sense that this Court shouldn't interfere with the processes of a state court unless it clearly appears that the constitutional rights of a defendant have been invaded somewhere during the course of his trial, and the burden is on the petitioner to show by a preponderance of the evidence that his constitutional rights have been violated in such a way that his trial was fundamentally unfair and he's been denied due process of law in the state courts.

"I might say I don't believe that the burden of proof has been sustained in this case. I don't believe a showing has been made here which would justify my releasing this petitioner, and I'll not spend very much time discussing my reasons. I think he was represented by counsel. I haven't the whole record here, but I have a number of excerpts, quite a substantial portion of it, and I think that his counsel, Mr. Selden, was competent and serious and alert in guarding the rights of this man and cross-examining the witnesses, particularly Officer Hickey, very vigorously, and I thought showed that he was doing a lawyer-like job in the defense. As I intimated in discussion with Mr. Bird, I can't believe that a judge who appointed counsel to defend a man would permit him to get up and try to help convict him and let that sort of thing go on.

"As to the change of venue, I have very little here to show that a fair trial was impossible in Pierce County. I know that the prospective jurors would be examined; they would be examined as to what they knew about the circumstances of this offense, what they had heard on the radio or read in the newspapers, and they would have to say, at least, that they had no preconceived opinion as to the guilt or innocence of the defendant, or have any prejudice against him. It's true that there is a good deal of feeling when an offense of this kind has been committed, but if the change of venue had been granted the case would have gone, under the state law, to an adjoining county, Thurston or King, and a case as widely publicized as this, I think the public would have known about as much about it in Seattle or Olympia, and whatever prejudice there may be against a man of the colored race, and I don't think that is very pronounced out here in the State of Washington, but whatever it might be would be just as existent in Thurston and King Counties as it would be in Pierce. Furthermore, the question of change of venue was fully argued to the Superior Court on arguments of counsel and affidavits and was one of the questions considered by the Supreme Court of the State, and the Supreme Court decided the motion had been properly denied.

"Now, as to the matter of the confession, I have carefully read all of the record that has been submitted here. Officer Hickey *did* admit that he physically mistreated this accused shortly after his arrest. It's an unfortunate incident, one that shouldn't occur in the administration of American justice, but Officer Hickey did offer an explanation for it, and it seems to me that it wasn't a part of a concerted scheme to coerce this man into making a confession. It was rather the sporadic and impetuous action of a man who was perhaps not too experienced in police work, and had been unduly influenced by a very ghastly sight that he had just witnessed and lost control of himself. That was the explanation given and it seems to me Hickey's testimony was frank. While he was reluctant to testify to what he had done, he did admit it, and it seems to me that if it had been a part of a police scheme, it would be easy to say, 'All the wounds were incurred while we were trying to arrest him,' and a number of them were. He was more severely injured, according to the police testimony, than he's said.

"I have tried to keep an open mind. I have tried to listen impartially to Mr. Bird's testimony, but the fact remains I do not fully credit his story that he was beaten for eight hours by a relay of police officers who were kicking him, stamping him and beating him with their clubs. He couldn't possibly have been in the condition in which Dr. Rickles found him at 11 o'clock the next morning. He would have been at the hospital in a hospital bed, it seems to me.

"Of course, the thing I'm concerned with here is whether or not the confession was voluntary or was coerced as a result of fear and intimidation at the time it was made, 11 a.m. the next day, and as against the testimony of the defendant that it was induced by fear and as a result of intimidation brought on by these beatings, we have the testimony of five other witnesses—Dr. Rickles, Lt. Lyons, Peterson, Deputy Prosecutor Mann, and Notary Public Anderson—that the confession was wholly voluntary, and as against the testimony of Mr. Bird I'm inclined to credit their written testimony and affidavits. And so the petition for Writ of Habeas Corpus will be denied, and the motion for stay of execution likewise is denied."

Time Runs Out

BY now, time had just about run out on Jake Bird.

With one foot in the courtroom and the other in the grave, his execution was penciled on the hangman's calendar for May 27, just five more days.

Playing it for all it was worth, Jake had one more legal maneuver up his sleeve. It was called a "Certificate of probable cause for appeal to the Court of Appeals in San Francisco."

On the fifth day, only 12 hours before he was to die, the Ninth Circuit Court of Appeals in San Francisco granted Jake a 30-day stay to determine whether or not an appeal could be heard. This marked the third time since his conviction that he'd been spared. "The gods are on my side," Jake said, self-righteously.

An *AP* news dispatch out of San Francisco explained:

> Judge William Denman of the Ninth Circuit Court granted the stay after receiving a petition from Bird. The brawny black contends his confession in the Tacoma slayings was forced from him by third-degree tactics.

> Judge Denman said the Circuit Court will hold a hearing in 10 days to determine whether a certificate of probable cause shall be issued. Such a certificate must be issued before the court can entertain an appeal.
>
> Previously, Bird had steered his case to a dozen courts, including the United States Supreme Court—twice—in an effort to gain an appeal.

On June 8, Chief Judge William Denman of the Ninth U.S. District Court of Appeals handed down his decision: *Appeal denied.*

Back in his cell at Walla Walla, the normally loquacious condemned man was strangely silent. When told of the judge's decision, all he said was, "Well, that's too bad."

Judge Denman held with three previous courts that there was no basis for Jake's complaint that police had beaten a confession out of him.

"I find no exceptional circumstances," Judge Denman wrote, "since the federal issue before the State Supreme Court and the U.S. Supreme Court was determined on the same evidence of claimed coercion as before the district court in Washington State."

There went the ball game. Jake had taken his case as far as it would go. He'd exhausted all the courts on his plea of coercion. Unless—miracle of miracles—he was able to gain new hearings on some other argument, his days in court were over.

Except for one.

He still had to appear once more in the original trial court in Tacoma to have his execution date fixed for the third time. All told, it would mark the 14th appearance in court for Jake in connection with his various appeals.

Deputy Sheriff Dave Ward, of Pierce County, was sent to Walla Walla to pick up Jake and drive him back to Tacoma. Davey was a former welterweight boxing contender—winner of 44 of 45 professional fights before World War II—and protege of World Middleweight Champion

(1936-38) Freddie Steele. Jake had better not get slippery with *him.*

From Walla Walla to Tacoma, the distance is about 300 miles—in 1949, a five-seven hour drive, depending on the driver's speed. Deputy Ward was bent on bringing Jake back as quickly as possible. Floorboarding it, he hit speeds of 80 and 90 all the way.

What was Jake's mood coming back?

"Talkative," Davey told me. "He talked up a storm."

About what?

"I asked him if he had any regrets about the people he killed. Only one, he said. He regretted having snuffed out that little boy back in Omaha who called him a nigger. He lost his head, he said. He confessed he shouldn't have done that. It was the only one of his murders he seemed remorseful about. He also told about a fight he had with a train detective in a boxcar. The door flew open, Jake pushed him out; he rolled underneath the wheels—and was cut in half.

"Death was old hat to Jake. He showed very little conscience. There was no predicting how many more people he'd have killed had he not been caught in Tacoma. However, he did say he wished he'd used his life in a more useful way. He was born and baptized a Catholic, he said. 'I didn't pay any attention to the teachings, though,' he said. 'I should have. My life would have been different.' I asked him about his family. He wouldn't talk about them. But he did want to talk about his hex magic. He said he'd put a hex on both Dr. Larson and Pat Steele. A double whammy. They'd die soon, sure as hell, he said. Just like the others. I said Steele was Irish and that you can't hex an Irishman. Jake said, 'Well, he's one Irishman I can hex, 'cause his ass is on backwards.' Jake hadn't lost his sense of humor.

"Every once in a while, Jake asked me to slow down. This was his last trip to Tacoma, he said, and he wanted to enjoy it. Every restaurant we passed, he'd say, '*Please,* let's stop and get some chicken.' At Yakima, I stopped to gas up and go to the restroom. I asked Jake if he wanted to relieve himself. He said no. But when we got on the other side of Yakima, in all that sagebrush country, he asked me to stop the car. Nature was calling, he said. I ignored him. I sensed what was going on inside his head. Despite the shackles binding him, he was planning to make a break for it, hoping I'd shoot him in the back and end it then and there. He'd have preferred that to hanging. I didn't give him a chance."

Deputy Ward asked Jake if he thought he would go to hell.

Jake said, "There is no such place. If there's a God, I'll get my punishment—but it won't be forever."

The signing of the death warrant was held in Judge Hugh Rosellini's court. The judge looked down at Jake and said, "Mr. Bird, do you have anything to say before I sentence you to hang and sign this death warrant?"

Jake rose from his seat. There was an air of dismay about him. What an actor, what a superb performance! He shuffled around in front of the bench and looked up at the judge with disbelieving eyes.

"Do I have anything to say?" he said. "You're asking me, *do I* have anything to *say?* Your Honor, I have quite a bit to say."

He let that sink in, then—

"First, I'd like to point out to your Honor that this affidavit you had me file—*you had me file this affidavit*—you said you would consider it. Well, the least you could've done is taken a recess and gone and read it. But, no, you didn't."

Jake turned to the crowded courtroom.

"And to you the people," he said, "I want you to know that this is just part of the road blocks barring my way to Olympia and all the way to the Supreme Court of the United State. This is the sort of thing—"

Judge Rosellini came alive.

"Mr. Bird—Mr. *Bird!*" he cried, gavelling for order.

Jake plunged right on.

"Mr. Bird—Mis-ter Bird!" pleaded the judge. "Address the Court, Mr. Bird! Address the Court!"

Jake was thoroughly enjoying himself. He was having a ball. Dr. Larson and Pat Steele were on the verge of cracking up. Pat had attempted to save Judge Rosellini from Jake, but he had insisted on letting Jake have his day in court. It was no contest. Jake had the ball and wasn't letting go.

After a brief recess Judge Rosellini's chambers opened. He strode to the bench. He sat down. He took a pen. He signed the death warrant (the third time he'd signed one for Jake). Then, finishing with a flourish, he said, "God hath mercy on your soul!" With that, he disappeared back into his chambers—before Jake had an opportunity to continue with his act.

Jake had been standing alongside Pat Steele. He turned to Pat and said, "Is that in accordance to Remington's Revised Statutes?"

Pat fought back a smile.

"Well, Jake," he said, straight-faced, "that's the way it goes."

In the disposition of capital cases in the United States, the median elapsed time between sentence and execution was for years approximately 17 months. In 1965 in Texas, an armed robber was electrocuted one month after his conviction; but in Louisiana that same year, two rapists had been waiting for a record 12 years. The variance depended a little on luck and a great deal on the extent of litigation. Jake Bird? The elapsed time between his original sentence and execution was about 20 months.

One crime reporter asked, "Has Jake Bird's travels through the many courts been an example of democracy at work—or a travesty on justice?"

At least one jurist in the case was inclined to take the latter viewpoint. In writing a dissenting opinion that Jake had filed a valid note of appeal, Judge Millard of the State Supreme Court said: "The majority opinion in effect says the more atrocious the crime, the more lax will be the rules of practice and procedure in favor of the criminal. Bird was entitled to a fair trial. He had a fair trial. The people are entitled to expeditious administration of justice in criminal cases."

Superior Judge Hugh Rosellini offered a broader view. In sentencing Bird to death, he urged Bird to find his salvation in God and then added: "Many persons not familiar with the legal workings of this case have been critical of its long delay. This has been to enable you to have every recourse to law. Despite the fact you are a member of a minority race, despite the fact you are penniless and unable to afford counsel, you have been before the state Supreme Court three times to argue your case. Unfortunately, Mr. Bird, the truth is not in you."

Jake Bird tugged at his neck.

The noose was growing ever tighter.

"The Lord Taketh Away"

PAT Steele was among the 50 or so witnesses who attended the hanging of Jake Bird, truly a *gallows bird* ("n: a person who deserves hanging"—Webster).

Dr. Larson did not go.

In France and Germany during the war, he had officiated at a few hangings. The way with that was this:

"I was stationed under the platform, which was covered with a black crepe cloth material," Dr. Larson said. "I stayed there waiting for the doomed man to drop through the trapdoor. God, it was awful. I mean, this terrible cracking noise of broken neck bones—like a leg of mutton mashing through a grinder. I'd wait for a few moments, letting him swing, then walk up and put the stethoscope to his chest. In hanging cases, the heart doesn't stop beating immediately. Sometimes it'd be five to ten minutes before I pronounced a body dead. A body goes through the damnedest contortions—like when you cut off a chicken's head, it does some wild things before dropping over. Well, a man who has just dropped and is dangling at the end of a rope goes through the craziest contortions. It's no fun to watch, I can tell you."

But for Steele, this was his first hanging—and he'd never forget it.

When Pat entered the death room at Walla Walla and saw the gallows, with its pale noose attached to a crossbeam, his heart skipped a beat.

"The room was quite large, like an auditorium," Steele told me recently. "The scaffold was in the forward part of the room with the traditional trapdoor. Howard Applegate, a stringer for *United Press,* was with me; so was Harold Stribling, one of Jake's earlier victims at Carter Lake, Iowa. Harold still carried a metal plate in his head where Jake had clubbed him. For 22 years, he had waited to watch Jake hang. He had lived all those years in fear that Jake would get out of prison and come back and kill him. At the trial, Jake had warned Stribling: 'I'll get you wherever you go.' And Stribling and his wife believed him. So there stood Harold alongside me at the Walla Walla gallows to watch Jake drop through that trapdoor."

At one minute past midnight, July 15, 1949, Jake Bird walked out of a side door directly onto the scaffold. He appeared calm. Any nervousness during the day had been disguised by a steady stream of conversation to almost anyone who would take the time to listen. He had still held out hope that his execution would once more be stayed by some official action. But that hope began to dwindle as night approached. First, the rejection from the United States Supreme Court, then the board of prison terms and paroles' hands-off attitude and finally word from Governor Arthur Langlie that he would not intervene. Toward evening, Jake told his attorney, Murray Taggart, that he could be a good loser if he knew everything possible had been done. And in all the records of criminal cases in the United States, no man probably had had access to more courts than Jake Bird.

During the afternoon, Jake had made out the menu

for the traditional last meal. It included fried chicken, two bananas, strawberries, ice cream and some orange soda pop. He also asked for two "black cigars."

His final requests were few. In a moment of irony he discussed a little black box but left his worldly possessions, $6.15, to his court-appointed attorney, Murray Taggart.

Accompanied by Warden Tom Smith and a prayer-murmuring Lutheran minister, Jake entered the death place handcuffed and wearing an ugly harness of leather straps that bound his arms to his torso. Warden Smith tried to help Jake as they walked out, and while his arms were pinioned, Jake shook the warden's arms loose. He could walk to the death place by himself, thank you. He took his position right on the trapdoor and waited for the noose to be slipped around his neck. His face was as blank and bland as ever.

Then the warden read him the official order of execution, a two-page document; and as the warden read, Jake's eyes, enfeebled by almost 30 years of cell shadows, roamed the little audience. As was customary, the warden, having finished his recitation, asked the condemned man whether he had any last statement to make. Jake remained silent.

"I have Mr. Bird's last statement," the minister said, and he began reading from a prepared paper. "The Lord giveth, the Lord taketh away. Blessed is the name of the Lord," the chaplain intoned as the noose was fitted and as a delicate black mask was tied around Jake's eyes. "May the Lord have mercy on your soul." The trapdoor suddenly opened, and Jake Bird hung for all to see a full 14 minutes before the prison doctor at last said, "I pronounce this man dead." A hearse, its lights blazing, drove up to the back door, and the body, placed on a litter and shrouded under a blanket, was carried to the hearse and out into the night.

Staring after it, Pat Steele shook his head: "I hate to see an old adversary go. But it's about time. I've seen all of him I want to see. He was a tough old boy to put down. I'm glad it's over."

Howard Applegate, the *U.P.* reporter, never saw Jake hang. Oh, he was there, all right, but he had been standing engrossed in his notes as the Lutheran minister read Jake's last statement, and when he looked up, there was Jake swinging by the neck. He never even heard the trapdoor spring open, so lost was he in his notes. He turned to Steele and said, "Pat, what happened?"

Pat Steele pointed to the swinging body and said, "There he is right there, Howard. You missed the hanging of Jake Bird."

The Phone Rings . . .

WHEN a forensic pathologist first starts working on homicide cases, it is understandable that he will have moments of queasiness. All of us, except undertakers I believe, have an instinctive negative reaction to death. The fact of death in its simplicity, however, is not what a forensic pathologist dealing in homicide must face. He must face the fact of death in all of the brutal horror of dismemberment, violation, decomposition and mutilation, for the bestial fury of man lashed to the point of killing knows no bounds.

Before one's breakfast it is somewhat unsettling to be called to a bus station or a railroad station to extract a dismembered body from three lockers—the legs and arms in one, the torso in a second and the head, carefully wrapped in newspaper, in the third. Especially when the attention of the transit authority who called had been generated by the heat of an early August morning. Also, a torso will swell as time goes on, quite filling the locker and annealing itself to it until pried loose with, let us say, a flat shovel.

Down the years there have been times when Dr. Larson has found his mind drifting from a death scene and wondering if he was really looking at what he *was* looking at; in one case, a man in women's panties with a brassiere strapped tightly to hold two tennis balls against his chest. He was hanging dead from a ceiling with a rubber tube connected in series, by the aid of pipettes in rubber corks, through a bottle of brandy, a bottle of ether solution and a bottle of soda water—to the urethera—the passage through his penis. With the other end of the tube at his lips, he had been blowing the mixture into his bladder when death took him.

A little investigative reading will straighten out the matter for you. Dr. Larson (and he has photos he has personally taken to prove it) has had cases where deviates have discovered that an *almost* hanging—that is, a suspension of the body by the neck not *quite* to the point of inducing unconsciousness—intensifies the pleasure of orgasm. Of course, some never lived to tell about it. In the case of the man in the brassiere and panties, was it murder or suicide? Neither. It was *accidental* death. The noose had slipped and strangled him before he could get himself stoned—and to the point of climax.

In the larger cities of America, homicides occur almost every day, although some of them are not highly publicized. The Dr. Larsons of the profession always have a backlog of cases. Dr. Larson could be busy all the time, if he wanted. Homicide investigation requires discussion and imagination and sometimes 24 hours of work a day, seven days a week. When a detective is working a case, there is no such thing as hours. The overtime buildup is so fantastic that it is almost ridiculous to keep track of it.

A good forensic pathologist, therefore, must be completely in control of his life, as far as working hours are concerned. Like Dr. Larson, he must be a man with highly developed curiosity. He has to like puzzles. A puzzle has to *bother* him. Some people can look at a crossword puzzle, or problem, fool around with it until it bores them and drop it. A good homicide man like Dr. Larson *can't*. He must have a nature wherein the puzzle itself captivates him, wherein it finally gets so far under his skin that he can't eat, he can't sleep. *He has to know the answer.*

He must have an orderly and a disciplined mind. He must not get *ahead* of himself, for if he does he is liable to miss a trick—a small but important movement in the game. For that is exactly what the working of a homicide is: a five-movement game. First, by a very thorough examination of the murder scene *when, where* and *how* are partially established. Those three elements are then frozen into the record for continual future reference by diagrams and dozens of photographs before the body is moved. *How* is completed by the autopsy report, and identification of the victim should begin to answer *why*. When you determine *why*, you have the motive. When you have the motive, you begin slowly to reach out for *who*.

The phone rings . . .

Some 120 miles west of Tacoma General Hospital, while investigating an untended bonfire on the beach near Ocean Shores, Washington, local police smelled gasoline in the night air. Within the burning driftwood, a deputy spotted a foot sticking out. Closer inspection revealed the badly charred body of a young woman. Weight was estimated, under preliminary examination, as approximately 110 pounds, height 5 feet 2 inches, about 23 years of age. Her face had been burned virtually beyond identification. Her clothing was mostly gone, burned, so there were no labels or laundry marks to help find out who she was. Dental examination disclosed only two ordinary amalgam fillings and three missing teeth. Unremarkable possibilities for identification.

The mystery called for a specialist.

The local police chief put in a call to Tacoma General and asked to speak to the Crime Doctor . . .

Dr. Larson's autopsy of the woman came up with five knife stabs in the body, two of which were undoubtedly the cause of death—one cutting into the heart and then going through and through the left lung. There were no soot stains in the mouth or the tracheobronchial tree (the throat and lung tops) which indicated that the girl had been dead *before* her body was placed in the fire.

"This was a very interesting case, a very *unusual* case," Dr. Larson said. "It's a classic illustration of how careful a forensic pathologist must be, or he'll never identify a body. But getting down to the examination, I did a very meticulous autopsy on the girl. There is no body so badly decomposed or burned that it does not deserve an autopsy. The tiniest clues often will pop up as important leads. I have had severely burned bodies—in fact, when practically nothing was left—and I was still able to determine, in some instances, the cause of death and even who the victim was. Once, just such a case led us to the killer, who was arrested and sent to prison. So it pays to be painstaking in the autopsy room.

"Actually, it's quite simple for a pathologist to determine the *cause* of death. That isn't the important factor in medical-legal cases. The important factor is to determine the circumstances surrounding a violent death. The manner of death. How did it occur? This will usually lead you to the murderer. Now, in the case of a shooting, any damned fool can tell you that a bullet went through the heart. That doesn't tell you very much, unless you know the *direction* of the slug, how far away the gun barrel was when fired, whether it was suicide or homicide, the elevation of the weapon when fired—all the hundred and one ancillary factors that a forensic pathologist understands and can pinpoint. Caliber of gun, type of gun the bullet was fired from, which is the bullet wound of *entrance* and which is the bullet wound of *exit*; all these things are determined by the forensic pathologist. On the other hand, an ordinary pathologist could probably tell you that the victim died of a bullet wound through the heart, but really, what does that tell you? It doesn't solve the murder for you.

"Well, you are probably thinking, what about fingerprints? In the case of the charred girl, her hands were practically burned off. No fingerprints could be obtained from the left hand, but the right hand gave us a scant few. However, most women in their twenties are not fingerprinted. Did you know that? There's no file kept on them. Consequently, we had no prints of her either at city or state identification departments. The FBI files didn't have any. That's one of the weaknesses in our system. There is no national fingerprint law. People have advocated such a law for years, but Congress has been reluctant to pass one—something about invasion of rights and privacy. Therefore, not everybody in the U.S. is fingerprinted. Only about half our country's population has fingerprints registered.

"Feeling that her fingerprints would only lead to a dead end, I next looked for fingernails. Sometimes you can make out a body from fingernail clippings. They never change and they're almost as accurate a form of identification as fingerprints. When you put them under a microscope and look at them in cross section, the lines and striations will match up identically with the fingernail from which they were clipped—even 10 years later, because no two people have exactly the same fingernail lines and striations. Yes, fingernails are very important. Unfortunately, the body I had was wearing *false* fingernails, which wasn't much help in tracking down the identity of their owner.

"With a body before you, you have, in most cases, every piece of the puzzle that is to be solved. A forensic pathologist must not *fail* to examine every possibility; to run down every indication until the truth is plain. Careless work on the part of investigators is the cause of failure to solve most of the backlogs of homicide cases that are piled up in every police department in this country.

"To the outsider, performing a thorough and careful autopsy is quite possibly not the tastiest dish of tea, but to me, it is always a silent challenge, and each one offers a completely new problem which it is my business to solve. Performing an autopsy is completely impersonal; reduced to a discipline that has, with the years, become so all-inclusive with me as to eliminate most of the possiblilities of failure. Personality disappears entirely with death, and all that remains is a laboratory specimen to be clinically examined with complete objectivity."

It dawned on Dr. Larson that the girl's death might have been sex-related. He examined her vaginal tract to see if she had been raped or assaulted. She had had recent intercourse, but there was no evidence of rape and she had no intact hymen. The doctor concluded that the fact she'd recently had intercourse was really insignificant. What *was* significant were the five stab wounds in her chest. One of them had slashed through the left ventricle of the heart, cutting across the septum. She had died very suddenly. The burning was all postmortem. The girl was dead *before* being stuffed in the fire. All the killer was doing was trying to destroy the evidence.

As Dr. Larson worked over the body, he remembered a snatch of something he had read once: "Murder is an abhorent crime from which God turns his face."

Nothing was more abhorent than what he had here.

Then it all opened up very fast. The charred lids of the girl's closed eyes were parted, revealing the fact that she was wearing contact lenses.

"The lenses were a bit disfigured by the heat of the fire," Dr. Larson remembered, "but clear enough to be examined. The fact that her eyelids were closed had saved the lenses from total destruction. Finally, we had our first big lead."

Under close scrutiny, Dr. Larson noted that the left lens had a blue dot in it; there was no such blue dot in the other but when examined under ultraviolet light a distinct "J" appeared. Curious, he started calling some ophthalmologists he knew in the area. He also phoned several optical supply houses specializing in contact lenses. He learned from them that the lens with the blue dot was manufactured by the Wesley Jensen Company, a Seattle firm. No supplier in Tacoma sold that particular brand, but there were a few Seattle outlets that did.

Dr. Larson again:

"I took the lens to an ophthalmologist who had all the proper equipment to measure them, and together with an occulist who worked for him, they did a thorough job. They measured the bevel on the lens, they measured its thickness, they determined all its features. On the basis of their answers, I started phoning every optician in Seattle—but to no avail. Then I started in on Burien. Bull's-eye! I found an optometrist who handled Wesley Jensen contact lenses. I gave him the prescription, he went through his files and came up with a name: a Burien ophthalmologist, Dr. Underwood, had prescribed just such lenses a year and a half before. I was certain I was on the right track."

Dr. Larson contacted Dr. Underwood, whose prescription for the contact lenses was compared to the wear-distorted lenses found on the eyes of the body. The manufacturing tolerance (that degree to which the actual lenses may vary from the prescription) for the magnifying power of the lenses was 0.125. Wear and exposure to heat will change certain factors in contact lenses. These were the factors which actually differed most between the prescription and the actual lenses. Finally, the lenses from the eyes of the body were studied by the technician who had made them—and identification became positive.

"So now we had the girl's name," Dr. Larson said. "We phoned her family, and yes, their daughter was missing.

She was married, no children. Roughly the body approximated the young woman's description. The daughter's husband was a prime suspect. We arrested him, and after an extensive investigation of all the physical facts, he broke down and made a full confession. This, then, was a case of assault, with very little evidence to lead us. What made it so special was that it marked the first time where a murder was solved on the basis of positive body identification from *contact lenses.*"

Dr. Larson and Hollis Fultz working together found that 95 percent of the murders of wives prior to 1945 were committed by husbands. When husbands are murdered, the wife, in some cases, has done the job, but murder, in spite of Women's Lib, is not a general occupational hobby of the female.

"She gets back in other ways," Dr. Larson says. "But again I must point out that the majority of homicides have a sexual connotation. That may range all the way from a Krafft-Ebing distortion of normality to a strong desire to change partners in midstream."

The phone rings . . .

In the Tacoma area some years ago, a householder was digging into the floor of his cellar to prepare a concrete base for a new staircase when his shovel began to turn up bones and fragments of disintegrated cloth. The police boxed the exhibits, including a skull with the lower jaw still in place, and brought them in to the Tacoma General Hospital lab for examination by Dr. Larson.

The top of the skull was fractured by a through-and-through bullet wound of entrance and exit. It was estimated by the extent of damage it had done that the bullet was either a .25 or .257 or a 30-30 caliber rifle bullet.

Pelvic examination bones indicated that the remains were those of a male, and examination of the arm and leg bones indicated that he had been a muscular individual, probably a laborer, and that he had, in life, been about 5 feet 5 inches tall. X-ray examination disclosed that he was between 30 and 45 years of age at death.

A picture of the victim was now beginning to form so clearly that at least an outline of the deceased could be drawn. To frame the picture, it was estimated that the bones had been buried at least 10 years, but no maximum date of internment could be set.

Armed with what Dr. Larson could give them, the police traced all previous owners of the house where the bones had been found and eventually reached a woman who 27 years before had moved out of the house and into another one two blocks away. According to neighbors, she had had at the time a common-law husband who'd gone to Alaska and had not returned, so far as was known. She had a son presently serving with the army in Korea. With the cooperation of federal authorities, her son was interrogated. At the age of six, he told investigators, he remembered his "father" coming home one night "as drunk as a skunk," as he put it, "and whaling the living daylight" out of his mother. In a lull in the action, his mother had told him to go to the closet and get the rifle. He had done so and his mother had shot the man. Together they had buried him in the cellar.

Thus, under careful and well-qualified examination, murder will out—even after 27 years.

Understandably, the woman got off with probation.

"I once had a case up at Neah Bay, Washington, where the bones of ten complete bodies were stumbled upon by hikers," Dr. Larson recalled. The sheriff up there wanted to know if it was a mass murder. After piecing together all the facts, I came to the conclusion they had died in an Indian war—that the bones actually were between 300 and 500 years old. I found antique weapons around the bones. The evidence indicated an Indian burial ground, and most of these people had been killed in battle. Of course, there was no dental work to help me in identification—they didn't have dentists in those days. The shape of an Indian's skull is slightly different from that of a white man's. In fact, a skull often will tell you whether it belonged to an Oriental, Indian, black or white. That's not always totally true, but almost, because the configuration of the skull differs from group to group. Teeth are another indicator. Indians, for example, wear their teeth *down*. An X-ray of the choppers will also give you an accurate estimate of age. At Neah Bay I found that one of the skulls had been fractured by a bone spear made out of animal bone.

"The ten skeletons went on record as victims of an ancient Indian war. We never could be positive about who they really were. Today, however, I could send such discoveries away to a lab and have them tested by Carbon 14 radioisotope studies. The technicians could probably come within 25 years of telling us how old those relics really were."

It must be borne in mind that Dr. Larson is not a mastermind detective, such as the fictionalized Perry Mason or Monsieur Poirot. Rather, he is a *scientist* whose work is performed mainly in the laboratory and whose conclusions are drawn scientifically from physical evidence gathered *from* and around a dead body.

And so—

The phone rings . . .

Backpedaling, some years ago the police up at Everett, Washington asked Dr. Larson for assistance. They had a head-scratcher on their hands. They had a body but no identification.

Dr. Larson:

The opening facts of the case were these: The body was female, about 26 years of age, 160 pounds, 5 feet 3 inches tall. She was found in the garbage dump by the garbage superintendent at 5 a.m. He was a natural suspect.

What in hell was he doing out there at 5 o'clock in the morning? She was dressed expensively but with conservative taste. Everything came, I'm sure, from the most fashionable shops in Seattle. Her shoes were off. They were found near the head of the body. Her girdle was pulled down, her dress was pulled up. The labels had been ripped off her garments. Semi-obese, there was blood oozing from her mouth. Acne covered her arms and face. When I arrived on the scene, her body was still warm. I estimated that she had been dead from six to eight hours; probably died between 10 p.m. and midnight.

Any time somebody tells you—or you see on TV or read in a James Bond novel—that whozis died at 11:10 p.m., don't you believe it! Nobody can be that accurate. Over the years I have learned through mistakes to leave a pretty wide margin when estimating how long somebody's been dead, especially if they've been dead more than 24 hours. After 24 hours and longer, you've got to take all the known facts into consideration—and then what you come up with is only an educated guess.

With the Everett girl, that wasn't the case, because she had only been dead a few hours.

We have many ways of telling how long a body has been cooling. One of the best means is to take fluid out of the eyes. The fluid is called aqueous humor, and you get it by putting a needle in the corner of each eye and drawing out about two milliliters.

This fluid can then be tested for various chemicals, including potassium. We normally know what the potassium level is, and we know how it increases each hour after death for at least the first 24 hours. We have a number of chemical tests that help us tell how long a person has been dead—fairly accurate tests, too. You can then measure the drop in body temperature and compare it with the temperature outdoors, and by knowing the clothing a person had on, you can make a pretty close guess as to how long ago the body stopped breathing. This can be done within reason, but after 24 hours it becomes a very difficult problem. Fortunately, most bodies are found before they have been dead 24 hours, so you don't face that baffling problem.

We noticed a lot of suffusion on the front of the young woman's neck—a lot of darkening of the skin—and that was due to the collection of blood from compression below that point. Usually that is a sign of strangulation, and I was almost certain she had been strangled to death. She had fingernail scratches on her neck. There were also marks where her girdle had been pulled down. They were fresh—and they were hemorrhages. That convinced me she hadn't removed or replaced the girdle herself. But somebody had—and *forcibly.*

The identification of this woman was fascinating. External examination showed widely dilated pupils, a protruding tongue, and there was an old surgical incision slightly to the right of the midline of the lower abdomen. There was blood coming from the vagina, and surgical scars were prominent on the outer sides of both big toes.

An abdominal scar does not necessarily lead to an identification. You may circulate all the hospitals in any city and find dozens of abdominal operations listed, with nothing outstanding to indicate upon whom the surgery was performed. But surgical scars on the outer sides of each big toe indicate bunionectomies, that is, the surgical removal of bunions. If you question hospitals on bilateral bunionectomies in young women, you'll find them not too common.

Within hours after I identified those toe scars for what they were, the Everett police had the name of a young woman of 25 who, the year before, had gone through a double bunionectomy operation. Investigators turned up the fact that she was, at present, missing.

McCallum:

Dr. Larson's autopsy revealed not *one* but *three* causes

of death. The first was fatal air embolism. The initial post-mortem incision showed bubbles of air in many of the superficial and deep abdominal veins. Air was aspirated (sucked out by syringe) from the right auricle and right ventricle of the heart. The blood still in the right side of the heart was laced with foam and air bubbles. Thus death *could* have been caused by an air embolism (the introduction of air into the blood stream so that when it reaches the heart, it acts in interrupting the blood flow precisely like a solid body does in *blocking* the blood flow).

Incidentally, the woman had large breasts with deeply pigmented nipples which suggested pregnancy. Dr. Larson concluded that air had been introduced into the uterine cavity (the womb) and from there into the bloodstream by means of a catheter. His immediate secondary conclusion was that an inept attempt at abortion had been tried. This was supported by the discovery that the uterus held a male fetus of about six and a half months' fetal age, as indicated by the crown-rump measurement (from the top of the head to the buttock).

A second probable cause of death was suggested by those scratches and hemorrhages in the neck area. This was confirmed by the discovery of hemorrhages in the strap muscles of the neck. She had been throttled.

A third probable cause of death was a large bruise on the forehead with hemorrhage over the surface of the brain.

Dr. Larson:

The reason women having an illegal abortion get air embolism is because the veins of the uterus are markedly dilated, enlarged and under negative pressure, so it's easy to open up some of these veins in the performance of an abortion and air is sucked into the circulation. Air is compressible. Like the air in your automobile tire, you can put a lot of air into one tire by air compression.

Air is compressible, whereas blood is not. When the

heart beats, it forces liquid blood into the circulation. When you get air in your heart, the heart contracts and the air compresses. It doesn't go anywhere, so no blood gets into the system. That, of course, is why people die. It takes about 200 milliliters of air in the vascular system to cause death in a human being.

Small amounts of air do not cause death. There have been many medical-legal cases where people have been tried in court—there was one back in Illinois, where a doctor was accused of killing a lady patient who had terminal cancer. He admitted injecting 20 cc's of air into her because she was hopelessly ill. Twenty cc's of air probably wouldn't even cause the heart to miss a beat. I went back and testified at the trial for the doctor. He was acquitted. There were some noted pathologists who testified that she died of air embolism, but they were not *forensic* pathologists. They were not genuine experts. The doctor probably would have been convicted had he not secured real experts to tell the court what air embolism really does and how much air it takes to kill a person.

In Everett I sucked about 150 cc's of air out of the victim's veins, so I knew that was what caused her death. When I opened her heart, it was filled with tiny air bubbles.

Three causes of death. How in hell do you explain three causes of death? I don't think anybody but an expert could have figured it out. I was able to because of some previous experiments on dogs. The purpose of the tests was to determine how much air embolus it takes to kill a dog. The experiments were conducted in Tacoma General Hospital surgery. An anesthesiologist assisted me. On one occasion a dog that wasn't properly anesthetized got away from us after being injected with air and went berserk. We were able to see what an unanesthetized dog does when injected with enough air to kill it. The animal lived for about two minutes and went absolutely crazy. He was barking, squealing and howling. He ran all over the surgery, defecating and urinating. It took us hours to clean up. The chief surgical nurse came in the next morning, threw up her hands, and cried, "What in hell happened here? Don't ever bring another damned dog into my surgery."

Knowing what that dog did, I was able to reconstruct what had happened in the case of the Everett woman. A catheter had been put into her to produce an abortion, and the air got into her system. She probably rose up off the bed, screamed and hollered at the top of her voice, and went wild. Everybody got so frightened they panicked. Somebody grabbed her by the neck to control her, while somebody else hit her on the head. She'd have died of air embolus if they hadn't done this, but it really didn't make any difference. That explains the bump on her head. She got that when they slammed her back on the bed. Somebody knocked her out with a club of some sort to quiet her down. She was also strangled.

After we finally identified the woman, it didn't take long to crack the case. We learned that she had been going with a wealthy married man, a next-door neighbor. She lived in a very fine part of town with her parents—a very respectable family. We had our lead. We started investigating him and discovered that he had a friend with a camper. The two of them and a hired practical nurse took off in the camper for the garbage dump to perform the abortion. When the girl friend went into the frenzy and died, they got scared, dumped the body and beat it.

Some of the inequities of justice are illustrated by this case. Before the wealthy boy friend was brought to trial, he was released on bond. He was finally tried and, believe it or not, received a suspended sentence. He had hired a team of very good attorneys. I was very upset when I heard the outcome of the trial, because I had had a similar case the week before in Olympia. The same sort of death, too—of a girl who was married to the accused. The young man had hired a practical nurse, and together they had attempted an abortion. The nurse told him to blow in the catheter.

She explained it would kill the baby. He blew in the catheter, all right, but killed his wife instead. He rushed her to the hospital emergency room, but it was too late. The jury brought back a second-degree murder conviction, and the judge gave him a 20-year sentence.

The inequity of these two cases made me mad. I was extremely unhappy with the judge for giving the young man such a stiff sentence, and I protested to him in writing. The man in the almost identical Everett case got off practically scot-free. Because the Olympia man didn't amount to anything, didn't have any money or influence, he was given a harsh sentence; whereas the wealthy boy friend in the Everett case got a suspended sentence. That made no sense to me at all, especially in view of the fact that the Olympia man had brought his dead and legal wife to the hospital, while the other guy left the dead girl in a garbage dump.

McCallum:

Dr. Larson feels he was lucky in the Everett case. He was able to go straight to the scene. As we have tried to stress in this book, he sometimes will not accept a police case if he isn't called immediately. At the scene he can do many things that police officers, as good as they are, are not qualified to do. Dr. Larson will think of all kinds of angles that other investigators often miss. That's not because he wants to hog the whole show. An investigation of a homicide is a cooperative business. You must have the teamwork of well-trained policemen, well-trained identification officers, well-trained criminologists and a forensic pathologist. *Then* you have an almost unbeatable team.

Dr. Larson:

When a body is found inside a house, I instruct the police to lock up the place, phone me, and the wheels roll. Once on the scene, we work from periphery inward. We look for evidence as we go. The last thing we do is look at the body. When we finally do get to the body, we handle it very carefully, because we might want to come back and look for something around it that might help solve the case. We are always picking up trace evidence of one kind or another.

In my opinion, it is virtually impossible to enter a house, commit murder and then scram without leaving trace evidence behind. If you look hard enough, you'll find it: a strand of hair, a fiber of clothing, a fingerprint, *something*. It may only be a tiny, microscopic bit of trace evidence, but the killer will leave something to connect him with the crime.

And that's all we need.

In his quiet and modest way, Dr. Larson is leaving his mark on crime investigation. Even upon Scotland Yard, so fabled in whodunits, but actually as old shoe a police department as any. In the previously described Dr. Fry case, I mentioned Dr. Francis Camps, for many years Scotland Yard's forensic pathologist. Sir Francis had been called upon for a deposition by the insurance companies and so was on the other side of the fence. Nevertheless, he and Dr. Larson, laboring professionally in the same vineyard, so to speak, were good friends.

When Dr. Camps, after the first International Congress of Forensic Pathology in Belgium in 1957, showed Dr. Larson through the Laboratory at Scotland Yard, the Tacoman was appalled at the antiquated equipment with which the Yard was working. The appropriation for the Laboratory was about 1,000 pounds ($2,600) a year. In contrast, Dr. Larson's crime lab in Tacoma had items not available to Scotland Yard. They didn't even have an atomic absorption spectrophotometer or a modern gas chromatograph.

Medicine changes very rapidly, and equipment has to be replaced just as fast. A few years back, approximately ten years elapsed before techniques and procedures became completely outdated. Now, there is less than a five-year gap, and the time is rapidly approaching when that gap could be reduced to 12 months. This means that the techniques used *last* year could be horse-and-buggy procedures *this* year.

It was strongly suspected by the British Parliament that what happened in London was the result of a benign conspiracy between Drs. Larson and Camps. At Heathrow Airport, just before takeoff for the United States (so that he could say it all once and suffer no backlash), Dr. Larson held a press conference and blew the lid off, to headlines of:

"SCOTLAND YARD OUT OF DATE, SAYS AMERICAN"

"BRITISH UPSET"

"TOOLS TOO OLD, U.S. EXPERT SAYS"

"SHADES OF SHERLOCK HOLMES—JARRING, WHAT?"

"SCOTLAND YARD CRITICISM WAS PLANNED MOVE"

An *Associated Press* dispatch out of London reported the story this way:

> An American expert set sparks flying today by describing Scotland Yard, Britain's police headquarters, as out of date.
>
> Dr. Charles P. Larson, president of the College of American Pathologists, said the Yard is in danger of losing its reputation as the world's most efficient crime squad.
>
> His criticism, voiced before leaving for New York after an extensive tour of the Yard, was immediately taken up in British newspapers. The *Daily Mirror* demanded a government investigation into Dr. Larson's charges.
>
> Dr. Larson said: "I was abslutely amazed to see how outdated the Yard's scientific equipment is. My own private equipment at home is better. Despite the fact that it has first-class men who know their job inside out, its reputation is going to be lost unless it gets more and better

equipment. It is shattering to find the best crime squad in the world with such outdated tools . . ."

The *Mirror* asked: "Is the British government mean to the world's most famous police force? It is outrageous if the world's finest detectives have to work with old and blunted tools."

The paper called for a government probe to establish whether the Yard needs more money to modernize its equipment.

"I was the first president of the International Society of Forensic Pathology," Dr. Larson recalls, "and after the meeting in Brussels, was flying back to the United States by way of England. At the invitation of Dr. Camps, I visited Scotland Yard. I was told about the problems the Yard was having getting appropriations from the British government for the laboratory. On my tour of the Yard, I spent two days talking with the lab people. I asked them what they needed to bring their equipment up to standards. I encouraged them to talk about their special problems. They were very candid; no doubt about it, their lab had fallen behind the times. The government simply wasn't funding them enough to keep up with modern crime.

"Dr. Camps asked me to talk to the British press. I said I would, on one condition. The press conference would have to be held at the airport, just before I flew back to the States. The rest is documented history. At Newfoundland, where we stopped briefly for refueling, the front pages of all the London papers had played up my interview in bold, black type: WORLD FAMOUS PATHOLOGIST SAYS SCOTLAND YARD OUTDATED. The stampede was on.

"When I walked into my house 24 hours later, my wife said, 'God, what did you do in London? The phone has been ringing off the hook. You must have had a thousand calls. Parliament members, lawyers, prosecutors, reporters, transplanted Englishmen living here in America have been phoning. Everybody suddenly wants to talk to you.' She was really hot, because the phone kept her up all night.

"I started taking the calls. Pro, anti, or neutral, they all wanted to comment on my remarks about the Yard. Some of the Britishers felt I was pretty hard on their grand old police force. Others got much more personal. One shouted into the mouthpiece, 'You cawn't defame the Yaad like that! Why, for two bob, I'd come 'ight over tha' and show you what's for!' They blistered the hide off me, making me feel like the late Abe Pollock, who used to referee prizefights. One spring, Abe thought he'd combine refereeing with baseball umpiring. He started in the bush leagues and didn't survive the first season. 'I stood for everything,' Abe mourned. 'They stepped on my feet with spikes, they kicked me on the shins and they bumped me around. One day, in Fort Wayne, the crowd was after me. I didn't mind what they said or did, how many pop bottles they threw or anything. But right in the middle of the game this big dame walked down the aisle carrying a bull terrier on a shawl strap, dropped it over the front of the grandstand railing and yelled, 'SIC HIM!' That's when I quit.'"

But Dr. Larson had his cheerleaders, too. Like this letter from William B. Dolan, Jr., M.D., of Arlington, Virginia:

> Dear Charlie: You sure gave them hell in England! I thought you might be interested in this clipping from the Paris newspaper. I first heard it (your interview) being discussed by two Englishmen in a cocktail bar in the Excelsior Hotel in Rome. They agreed with you.

On Dr. Larson's next visit to Scotland Yard, it was more than mere coincidence that the lab sparkled with modern new equipment.

New Year's Eve celebrations do not always end on a happy note.

On the last day of 1959, Dr. Larson received a call from the police about a hit-and-run accident. The victim was a woman who was coming out of a tavern, and as she started across the street at 1 a.m., a car traveling at high speed hit her, carrying her half a block. No witnesses.

That was when Dr. Larson became involved.

"My first act was to perform an autopsy," Dr. Larson began. "That was what really cracked the case. It demonstrated once more why autopsies must be done on accident victims. The woman's death was due to a fracture of the skull and massive injuries to the brain. In examining the body for clues, I found a tiny chip of green paint which proved to be very important. Miniscule paint chips can be examined microscopically and spectrophotometrically. This may tell you precisely what kind of paint it is—even the make and year of car it came from. If the car had a repaint job, even that can be determined."

Dr. Larson took that paint chip, which had been embedded in the skin just below the victim's breast, and came up with the answer: It was from a 1956 Plymouth.

In less than a week, police detectives located the death car. The driver, a teenage boy, had attempted to cover up his tracks by replacing the smashed front headlight. He had even tried to fix the dented fender himself.

"The boy made a full confession," Dr. Larson recalls. "It was New Year's Eve. He was full of booze, in a hurry and didn't stop. The courts call this *negligent homicide.* The fact that he was drunk and probably didn't know what he was doing was no valid excuse for not stopping.

"Police blotters have sucked up a lot of ink on cases like this. It is important that they be solved. Negligent homicides should be punished. This acts as a deterrant to those who blatantly think they can get away with it. It is damn difficult to get away with a hit-and-run homicide. Often the car will leave telltale evidence on the victim—and, by the same token, the victim will leave evidence on the car, such as weave patterns, fragments of clothing or human tissue.

"I have had any number of cases where a pedestrian

has been hit, caught under the car and then dragged. The trick here is to find the hit-and-run vehicle quickly. You can always find human tissue or other evidence underneath the car which will help reconstruct what really happened. A thorough examination will *prove* that the car ran over a human body. That doesn't mean we will be able to prove necessarily whose body it was the hit-and-run car hit, but it is a beginning. Once we have linked up the death car with the body, we have our killer.

"Conversely, sometimes a person is accused of hit and run, when, in actuality, he is *innocent.* As an example, some years ago I was called to Stanford University to investigate a hit-and-run negligent homicide. Both the suspect and deceased had been living in a fraternity house on campus. The body was found on the street in front of the frat house. The suspect's car had a broken headlight. When questioned, he said he broke it weeks before. There were no witnesses. The police did not buy his story and arrested him. They took him to the county seat at San Jose and booked him.

"Lowell Bradford, the eminent criminologist who runs the lab at San Jose, had the suspect's car lifted on a hoist and examined underneath. He found blood. Unfortunately, that was as far as he went.

"When I was called into the case by the attorney for the parents of the accused boy, the first thing I did was to put the car back on the hoist. I found some blood and tested it in the lab. It was *not* human blood. It was *rabbit* blood. The suspect had been driving on the desert—jackrabbit country—and had hit a rabbit, splattering blood on the car's underbelly.

"If you use the correct antiserum, it is possible to establish what species of animal that unknown blood comes from. I have antiserums for most kinds of animal blood. There's a horse antiserum, for instance. Often the Health Department's meat inspectors call me in to determine if hamburger has been mixed with horsemeat. It's possible to tell even if only a tiny bit of horsemeat has been added.

"I love the story about the World War I soldiers who complained to their mess sergeant about the horse meat rations. The mess sergeant was unmoved. 'It's 50-50—chicken and horse,' he said. 'Yeah,' said the men. 'One horse and one chicken.'

"I have had several cases where two or three cars ran over a body. Say the body is prone in the road, having been struck down by car No. 1. It's a busy highway and car No. 2 comes along, strikes the body and doesn't bother to stop, either. He's afraid he'll get in trouble if he stops, figuring that the body was still breathing when he hit it. So he panics and speeds on. Then car No. 3 comes along and also runs over the victim.

"I had a case just like this, with three cars involved. The driver of car No. 3 braked his wheels just in time, however, to avoid hitting the body. He stopped, examined the body, and then called the police. Autopsy disclosed that two different cars had run over the deceased—at two different times. An examination of the cars told us which car hit the pedestrian first and which car had actually killed him. The impact of the first car hurled the victim into the air. He suffered all his fatal injuries when he hit the hood ornament and the windshield. Car No. 2 then ran over and pulled the body along. Legally, the second driver was not the killer because the body was already dead—from the impact of car No. 1. Both legs were broken at bumper-height.

"Driver No. 1 was convicted of negligent homicide, and Driver No. 2 was set free. This case demonstrates why automobile manufacturers have stopped embellishing the hoods of their cars with all those deadly weapons."

Police work differs radically in different parts of the country. Just as do criminals. Old cons, for instance, who have done Big House time in Arizona, Oklahoma and Florida will seldom pull a second job—at risk of a second stretch—in those three states, for the punishment there seems to be preventive.

There is a continual flow of outlander criminals through Los Angeles, Palm Springs, the Arizona sun towns and Las Vegas, but they use those places as resorts, not necessarily for capers. Ride the Sunset Strip in the nightly Intelligence car and you'll spot them from all over the country—the world sometimes—drinking, relaxing, wenching. These people have to be watched, reported upon to their home areas of activity and, as it were, shadowed off the premises.

Back in the late 1950s, Dr. Larson received a phone call from the Nevada State Patrol. It seems the NSP had a murder on its hands in Reno and had failed to come up with the answers. There had been three autopsies performed on the body—one by a pathologist—and still they were unable to list the cause of death. The police were stymied. *Please,* was Dr. Larson available? Dr. Larson made arrangements with the NSP as to what approach to the case he would take, adding that his fee would be $100 a day (in those days, that was considered a steep price). His terms were met and when he arrived in Reno, one of the local newspapers greeted him with these headlines: "OUTSIDE EXPERT CALLED IN—FEE $100 PER DAY." His *fee* had made the front page!

The case involved a young woman of 22, a Philadelphia heiress, worth about $5,000,000. By the time Dr. Larson took over the investigation, her estate had already hired a battery of Philadelphia lawyers.

Dr. Larson started slowly back over all of the information given to him by the NSP—picking holes here and building onto it there—but at second hand now—not with the fresh opportunity a properly trained homicide expert has if he is *first* on the scene.

Dr. Larson:

The girl was found murdered in a Carson City motel. A fascinating part of the case was her history. She had been a very well-known debutante. Her coming-out party had cost her parents upwards of $100,000 and was given a six-page spread in *Life* magazine. When she was 18, she'd married a lawyer from Philadelphia and four years later came to Reno for a divorce. She moved into a very posh place called the Happy Valley Ranch. It catered to wealthy ladies who were getting Nevada divorces.

I began my investigation there. It was everything the advertisements said it was—and more. Not only was it luxurious, with beautiful rooms and a lovely swimming pool, but the management had loaded its payroll with a good supply of handsome young men—*studs*. The guests were given their picks. Each woman had her choice of at least 20 young men, who would line up in front of her and let her choose which one she wanted for a roommate. It was all included in the $100-per-day package.

Our Philadelphia heiress selected a tall, bronzed, athletic chap—a typical love-for-sale Romeo. He moved in with her, and she quickly fell in love with him. That was her first mistake. The second was marrying him.

It turned out that the guy was a "paper-hanger" by profession. You know, a person who forges checks. He had a jail record. I think she knew this, but she married him anyway. Obviously, she was head-over-heels in love with him. In an attempt to reform him, she bought him a ranch north of Carson City and stocked it with fancy horses. She pampered him, gave him whatever he wanted. But still the guy was not satisfied. He still longed for his old profession. Paper-hanging was still in his blood, like a disease. It's one of those few crimes in which there's a tremendous recidivism. Consider the facts: He had all the money he needed, a new house, a new ranch and horses, a garage full of fancy cars—but he had this disease. Inevitably, he was arrested in Vegas for writing bad checks, and his wife bailed him out. He landed in jail a second time, and again she put up the bail. Then he went across the state line into California—supposedly on a "business trip"—and was nailed once more. This time his wife threw up her hands and told him, "To hell with you! I've bailed you out of jail for the last time! You can rot in there! I'm getting another divorce!"

Now the plot begins to thicken. She returned to Happy Valley Ranch and selected another stud out of the lineup. That proved to be the *coup de grace.* The next thing her friends knew, her body was found in a motel room in downtown Carson City. The room was registered to Stud No. 2. He was married, had two small children living in Massachusetts, and his wife had an arrest order out for him for nonsupport. He was a prime suspect. We could forget about Stud No. 1, because he was still in jail when the murder occurred.

You probably find it strange that the police didn't know *why* the heiress died, after three autopsies. Well, they didn't know because the autopsies were performed by people who weren't medical-legal pathologists. Consequently, they didn't know enough to do a careful dissection of the neck organs. So when I first saw the body, that's the first step I took.

According to the police, the body was found stuffed in a closet at the motel. A horrible stench indicated that it had been there for several days. The body was badly bloated and decomposed. The police showed me a sash cord which had been cut and had a knot in it. Incidentally, I should explain that during the fourth autopsy I found hemorrhages in the neck organs. X-rays also revealed a fractured bone in the neck. I was convinced that the cause of death was strangulation by a ligature.

I then took a sharp scalpel and scraped the sash cord. I found nothing, at first, but this was right after I started doing what is known as cytology, for the diagnosis of cancer, where we take a so-called pap smear of a woman's cervix and study it to decide whether or not a woman has cancer or is predisposed to cancer of the cervix or uterus. It was also right at that time we discovered you could take epithelial cells (found on the surface of the skin and the cervix), and with special staining, followed by microscopic examination, if the cells are from a female, you'll find what is called a Barr body in each one. Nobody but a female has Barr bodies.

I took this material off the sash cord, stained it, and lo and behold, I found cells very definitely with Barr bodies and very much female. I had proof, now, that the sash had been around a female's neck. That was a big break in solving the case. We also had the name of the fellow who had rented the room.

By now, Stud No. 2 had run off with the victim's car. We advised police across the country to be on the lookout for him. His wife in Massachusetts was also contacted. Damned if he didn't show up in her little town a week later to see her and the children. He was easy to spot, because he was still driving the victim's station wagon. The local police arrested him, and he was extradited to Reno, where he made a full confession and was sentenced for second-degree murder.

What made that case so special? Well, it was the first case that I know of that was solved on the basis of *cytology,* a brand new technique. It was a big boost for forensic pathology and just went to show that with the proper education anybody might solve such murders. An f.p.'s biggest assets are his imagination and perceptiveness. Of course, it helps if he has plenty of time to mull over a puzzle and think things out. You don't just rush into a tough case, because there is a danger of destroying evidence. You must have ample time to *think* a case out and use your imagination. There's really something to this Sherlock Holmes business, make no bones about that.

The best forensic pathologist is not necessarily the

most highly trained man. Rather, he's the man who uses logic and common sense. I very frequently let the police watch an autopsy, because with their curiosity and intelligence they often give rise to questions I don't think of and which are important. I've gotten a lot of education from inquisitive police officers peering over my shoulders in the autopsy room. I like having them there. In fact, I like to have them help conduct the whole investigation. When I first begin a case, I call in the police officers assigned to me and we have a conference. We review all the particulars and decide our strategy. Then we all begin to work as a *team.* At the scene we start at the entry door; we study it. If there's a screen on the door, if it's been cut—if there's been any disturbance, any marks of entry on the outside of the house—this is all recorded. We work our way in through the rooms of the house, examine everything as we progress, take pictures as we go, and collect trace evidence. I have a portable vacuum cleaner with a filter in it to pick up hair and particles so tiny you can't even see them with the naked eye. I later take the filter to my lab and examine all the contents. Attention to such detail often leads to important clues. A forensic pathologist is trained to know what to look for and what the evidence means. But if he fails to go to the scene, he is licked. I always insist on going to the scene.

After an inspection of the body and collection of the trace evidence, I have the victim removed to the mortuary, where a complete and exhaustive autopsy examination is conducted. Depending on the complexity of the case, this can take from one to ten hours.

At this point, everyone who has worked on the case retires to a place with a pleasant atmosphere, such as a bar-restaurant where we hold a post-autopsy conference and summation. I carry a dictating machine with me and record everything. I encourage all members of the team to express their opinions, ask questions and make suggestions as to how the case can be solved. What evidence do we have? What does the evidence *mean?* Everybody has an opportunity to get in his two-bits' worth.

One to three hours later I finish by telling the team what I will be doing in the laboratory. When the conference is over, we all have a pretty good idea where the case stands—what has been done and what is going to be done. Teamwork is so important! That's why we are able to solve so many cases, and why we have such a high percentage of solutions to homicides.

Summing Up

WHENEVER Dr. Larson uses the word "we," you are justified in reading it "I"—for the doctor is a personally modest and self-effacing man, dedicated to the "team" concept of investigative work. "A man never does the complete job alone," he says.

There is one hidebound rule, he stresses, that *must* govern a sleuth when he proceeds toward the solution of a crime: In every step he takes, he must follow a pattern of logic that is acceptable to more than one person. "It is a fact," he says, "that many men acquire this habit of mind through instinct, but the technique as a stipulated basis of procedure comes from the CIA in the beginning days: 'Don't work for yourself—be sure another mind is in agreement.'"

Because he has worked so closely with them for 40 years, the police have a special place in Dr. Larson's heart. "Policemen, by and large, are a very special breed," he'll tell you. "The average intelligence is far above the old days—and more honest. A dishonest cop is as rare today as a dishonest doctor. Straight out of the academy, I find them dedicated, eager to learn. Meet them halfway, and they'll work with you right down the line. They are good people to have on your side."

Dr. Larson is the first to tell you that when a man joins a police force, puts on the uniform, straps on the gun, this is in his mind: "Whatever you pay me, a hundred dollars a month or a thousand and a half, you now have a claim on my life. I am *your* gun, *your big stick."*

The early settlers along the frontier used to hire "guns" by their previous reputations. "Here are our laws—this is how we want our lives ordered. Come in and make it so." So the marshall and the western sheriff came into being—often starting their own lives elsewhere as outlaws—and as often as not redeeming themselves by ultimately losing their lives in defense of law and order at 20 paltry dollars a month.

"It isn't entirely the money that attracts a youngster to police work, even at today's relatively high-wage scales," Dr. Larson points out. "The motivating factor is not solely the pay. It couldn't possibly be. Remember, please, that unlike other men, the policeman leaves his home in the morning, kisses his wife goodbye, but each time he does it he knows by statistics that it may be the last time. Your efficient policeman, like your combat soldier, however, cannot be a brooder. He takes the risk in stride. He wasn't drafted, he asked for it, and a part of the asking was to dedicate himself to the proposition that anywhere, anytime that day, if a situation demands it, he will put his life on the line—for law and order—without the slightest hesitation. So in talking about the qualifications of a police officer, you have to go far beyond the mental, the physical and the medical tests. You have to get *inside* your man to find out whether he's the kind who can commit himself totally to such dangerous work. Fortunately, I have been able to attract people with that total commitment."

"Like Dr. Burton?" I asked.

"Yes," he said.

Until his recent retirement and move to Mercer Island in suburban Seattle, John F. Burton, M.D., was chief deputy medical examiner of Detroit and the County of Oakland, Michigan. Certified in 1949, he is the first *black* forensic pathologist in the United States—the *only* one in the country's history.

Drs. Larson and Burton first met in 1958 at a forensic pathology conference in Chicago. They have been good friends since.

Recently, during a visit at Dr. Larson's home, I asked Dr. Burton how he got started. He threw back his head and laughed heartily.

"Dr. Edward Zawadski, chief medical examiner of Detroit, told me that if I'd go down to the Detroit River and collect all the bodies that came to the top, he'd pay me $25 apiece," he said. "That was in 1949. There was an extra $5 per in it if I'd autopsy the heads."

Dr. Burton noted my eyes popping out like hard-boiled eggs.

"Listen," he said. "I was as poor as a church mouse. I needed the work—and the Detroit River was crowded with bodies. It was a popular dumping spot for the Mob."

Since it was his territory, Dr. Larson wanted to know what happened to Jimmy Hoffa.

"That's the most perplexing case I've ever had," Dr. Burton told him. "I got a call saying Hoffa had disappeared and for me to be prepared. Then I telegraphed five consultants and told them to get ready. We alerted all those people—got their plane fares ready—and then *nothing.* That's the end of the story. Oh, we spent thousands of dollars around his neighborhood in Pontiac, digging, scraping and excavating, trying to find Hoffa's body. But we got nowhere. Zilch. After a week everybody went home —and that, sir, ended the search for Jimmy Hoffa. Damnedest case I've ever known. His tracks ended at a restaurant. From there he just disappeared in thin air. Those people play rough. Every time I turned around, somebody from the Jimmy Hoffa clan was missing. He had a lot of enemies."

We were alone once more, wrapping up the loose ends of this book.

"I enjoy it all," Dr. Larson said. "The medical part, the police part. I even enjoy studying and researching malpractice cases. I'm curious to know whether there really has been malpractice, whether the treatment which a physician gave to a patient was really as poor as charged. If the answer is yes, then I'll testify for the plaintiff. I do a lot of case studies for the major malpractice insurance carriers in our state. A pathologist is peculiarly qualified to render a rather impartial opinion of the performance of another doctor, because he knows so much about the end results—what has happened, what can happen. His broad education in the medical-legal field is very helpful, especially if he specializes in medical-legal work, as I do. So in cases of malpractice, you can be a big boost to all parties—the insurance company, the accused doctor or the plaintiff. Very often you can advise the plaintiff and her physician that, in your opinion, there was no malpractice; that the accused doctor did a good job—that they are misinterpreting the whole thing. On the basis of that sort of consultation, very often they will drop the case."

He really enjoys going to court, he said. Being an expert witness, that's his cup of tea. But he doesn't go to court, he said, unless he is positive of his facts. He does not testify for the *money,* it goes deeper than that.

"It's like a game of chess," he said. "It's wits against wits—yours against an attorney's who is trying to upset you, to make you explode, to disqualify you and to make you look foolish in front of a jury. He may play every dirty trick in the book to win his case. But I have no fear when I get on that stand. I am not jittery. I love the challenge of cross examination. It's all part of the game."

There was once a well-known attorney in Tacoma who put Dr. Larson on the stand in an important case.

"Well, Dr. Larson," he said, "the prosecution consulted you on this case, isn't that true?"

"Yes," Dr. Larson replied.

"The prosecution is paying you—true?"

"Yes, sir."

"How much are you getting?"

"I charge by the hour. If you wish my standard rates, I'll be glad to give them to you."

"Well," continued the attorney, "when you investigate a case, you try to help the people who are retaining you, don't you?"

"Yes, if they deserve help."

"That's not exactly what I mean. I mean, you lean over backwards, and you try to find all the facts that will help the side that is employing you. Isn't that true, Dr. Larson?"

Dr. Larson straightened, leaned forward.

"Sir," he said, calmly, "I'm afraid you're confusing my profession with *your* profession."

End of cross-examination.

All through this book, there was a question I was burning to ask Dr. Larson. Is the perfect homicide possible?

"With a good forensic pathologist and a good investigative team working with you," he said, "I don't think there is such a thing as a perfect crime. The perfect crime only occurs when there's a poor investigation. In places where there is a qualified medical-legal investigative system, it's damned difficult to get away with murder. Unfortunately, more than 60 percent of the U.S.'s population is not served by a good medical-legal investigative system."

Dr. Larson has helped to establish the medical-legal investigative system in many states via the lecture platform. He even lectured to state legislators who were in hot debate over the question of adopting a medical examiner system. He has talked to community groups, doctors and all kinds of law enforcement organizations. After a lecture sweep through Texas, all the major cities of the Lone Star

State voted in the medical examiner system—Houston, Dallas, Galveston, Forth Worth and San Antonio.

"Shortly after a swing through Michigan," Dr. Larson said, "the legislature passed a law permitting counties of a certain size to have a medical examiner system. That included Detroit, which has had it for about 25 years now. California also has a good system. The coroner system. Actually, the coroners are appointed. Most of them are well qualified forensic pathologists. Florida has endorsed a similar program. New York has medical examiner systems in the major cities, but not in all the rural areas. Chicago has been noted for its inadequate medical-legal investigative system. They've never been able to get a good forensic pathologist to work there permanently because of politics. Pennsylvania has a permissible system, whereby the counties make their own rules and regulations."

And so we come to the end of the book.

"You got a good ending for it?" the doctor asked.

"Well, how's this?" he said. "There was this guy we'll call Artie. He was having a couple of beers with his pal Jules one night. Bolstered by the liquor, Jules told Artie he was damn sick and tired of his wife and sure would like to get rid of her. He said he'd pay Artie $1,000 if he'd choke her to death. Artie said, 'I don't like your wife, either. I never have liked her. Hell, I'll be glad to do it for a buck.' So Jules told Artie how to get into the house, the time to be there and how to choke his wife without getting caught. Artie followed the plan to the letter. He choked the wife and then, just as he was leaving the bedroom, he ran into the maid. To avoid leaving any witnesses, he choked her, too. Then the butler appeared—and he had to choke him, too. The next morning the newspaper headlines read: ARTICHOKES—3 FOR A DOLLAR!"

Appendix

Curriculum Vitae of Charles P. Larson, M.D.

Born: Eleva, Wisconsin, August 15, 1910.
Graduate: Gonzaga University, A.B. Degree, 1931; McGill University, Montreal, Quebec, M.D., C.M. Degree, 1936.
Internship: Pierce County Hospital, Tacoma, Washington.
Postgraduate training in Pathology: University of Michigan and University of Oregon Medical Schools.
Certified: in Pathologic Anatomy, Clinical Pathology, and Forensic Pathology by the American Board of Pathology. Certified by American Board of Legal Medicine.
Currently: Director Emeritus of Laboratories of Tacoma General Hospital, and co-owner of private laboratories in Tacoma, Washington. Five partners.
Member of following professional societies:

1. College of American Pathologists
2. American Society of Clinical Pathologists
3. American Academy of Forensic Sciences
4. Pacific Northwest Society of Pathologists
5. Pacific Northwest Society of Neurology and Psychiatry
6. American Psychiatric Association (Life Member)
7. American Medical Association

8. International Academy of Pathology
9. International Association for Identification (Life Member)
10. Law-Science Academy of America (Founding Member)
11. Law-Science Foundation (Founding Member)
12. Military Surgeons
13. Aero-Space Medical Society
14. Northwest Check Investigators Society
15. Inter-Society Cytology Council
16. La Asociacion Espanola de Medicos Forenses (Honorary Member)
17. Society of Medical Consultants to the Armed Forces
18. Association of Clinical Scientists
19. American College of Legal Medicine (Honorary Fellow)

Professional offices held:

1. Past President of Pacific Northwest Society of Pathologists, 1949.
2. President of North Pacific Society of Neurology & Psychiatry, 1949.
3. Member of Executive Committee, Washington Division of Mental Health Association, 1953-56.
4. Member of Executive Committee and Assistant Chairman of Executive Committee of Washington Division, American Cancer Society, 1940-58.
5. President, Washington Division of American Cancer Society, 1958-59.
6. President, College of American Pathologists, 1957-59.
7. Chairman of Council on Forensic Pathology for the American Society of Clinical Pathologists, 1957-63.
8. Chairman of Forensic Pathology Committee of College of American Pathologists, 1955-58. Developed certification program for American Board.
9. President of International Congress of Forensic Pathology, 1957-60.
10. Pathologist for War Crimes Investigating Team No. 6328, European Theater of Operation, March 1, 1945 - July 1, 1945.
11. Colonel, United States Army Reserve (Retired).
12. Commanding Officer, 359th General Reserve Hospital, 1949-64.

13. Vice-President, International Congress of Clinical Pathology, 1960.
14. President, Washington State Society of Pathologists, 1947.
15. President, McGill Graduates Society, 1952.
16. Board of Directors, National Committee for Careers in Medical Technology, 1953-59.
17. Member, AMA Committee on Legal Medicine, 1957-59.
18. Member, Executive Committee, Committee on Chemical Tests for Intoxication, National Safety Council, 1948 to present.
19. Vice-President, International Society of Clinical Pathologists, 1960-64.
20. Member, International Inter-Society Committee on Pathology for World Health Organization, 1956-62.
21. Forensic Medicine Editor, Medicolegal Digest, 1960.
22. Member, AMA Committee on Nuclear Medicine, 1962.
23. Consultant to American Board of Forensic Pathology.
24. President, Pierce County Medical Society, 1966-67.
25. Member, Board of Trustees, American Society of Clinical Pathologists, 1966-68.
26. Official representative of College of American Pathologists to AMA meetings, 1956-64.
27. Member, Board of Turstees, Pierce County Medical Bureau, 1965-67.
28. Vice-President, Washington State Medical Association, 1967-70.
29. Chief ASCP Councillor, World Association of Pathology Societies, 1969-72.
30. Member, Pierce County Hospital Council, 1971 to 1974.
31. President, Board of Governors, Lakewood General Hospital, 1970-76.
32. President, National Association of Medical Examiners, 1972.
33. Treasurer, Affiliated Hospitals of Pierce County, 1972 to present.
34. International "Inform" award in Forensic Pathology, 1967.
35. Distinguished Service Award, ASCP, continuing education.

Teaching positions:

1. Professor of Anatomy and Histology, St. Martins College, Lacey, Washington, 1939-41.
1. Instructor, Pathology Department, University of Oregon Medical School, 1940-42.
3. Assistant Clinical Professor of Pathology, University of Washington Medical School, 1948 to present.
4. Lecturer, Biology, University of Puget Sound, 1959.
5. Professor of Forensic Pathology (Visiting), University of Texas, 1959-63.
6. Assistant Professor of Biology, University of Puget Sound, 1959 to present.
7. Director of Approved Residency training program in Pathology.

Consultant positions:

1. Madigan General Hospital, 1946-77.
2. Western State Hospital, 1946-63.
3. Armed Forces Institute of Pathology, 1956-75.
4. Columbia University, Western consultant to Pathology Department, 1959.
5. M.D. Anderson Hospital and University of Texas, Department of Pathology, 1959.
6. Rayonier Marine Research Laboratory, Hoodsport, Washington, 1958-63.
7. Tacoma Police Department Crime Laboratory, 1946-75.
8. Veterans Administration Hospital, American Lake, Washington, 1958-77.

Scientific exhibits:

1. American Medical Association, 1939, 1940, 1947, 1954, 1955, 1956, 1957, 1958.
2. Numerous State and Regional Medical Society meetings.

Scientific papers: Sixty original papers written and contributed to American medical literature.

Civic activities:

1. Member, Board of Freeholders, City of Tacoma, 1954.
2. Chairman, Washington State Athletic Commission, 1958.
3. Member, Washington State Athletic Commission, 1959-65.
4. Rotarian (Since 1940).
5. Member, Board of Directors, Tacoma-Pierce County Blood Bank, 1946 to present.

6. President, Tacoma Athletic Commission, 1955.
7. Chairman, City of Tacoma Armed Services Committee, 1948.
8. Member, Washington State Advisory Committee on Mental Health, 1957-59.
9. Past President, Footprinters Boysville, 1952-55 (Branch of International Law Enforcement Association).
10. Surgeon General, Washington State AMVETS, 1949-53.
11. Medical Advisor, National Wrestling Association, 1960-63.
12. President, Washington State Junior Sheriffs Organization, 1961.
13. Reserve Officers Association, 1946 to present.
14. President, National Boxing Association, 1961-62.
15. First President, World Boxing Association, 1962-63.
16. Member, World Boxing Council, 1963.
17. Distinguished Service Medal, U.S. Army, 1968.

Index

D

E

F

G

H

I

J

K

L

M